5TH Edition

BEST ⋏ TENT
Camping

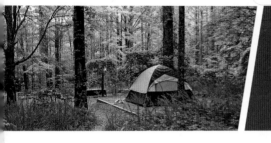

Southern Appalachian and Smoky Mountains

YOUR CAR-CAMPING GUIDE TO SCENIC BEAUTY, THE SOUNDS
OF NATURE, AND AN ESCAPE FROM CIVILIZATION

This book is for Keri Anne

Best Tent Camping: Southern Appalachian and Smoky Mountains

Printed in the United States of America
Published by Menasha Ridge Press
Distributed by Publishers Group West
Fifth edition, first printing

Library of Congress Cataloging-in-Publication Data for this book is available at catalog.loc.gov.
ISBN: 978-1-63404-149-2; eISBN: 978-1-63404-150-8

Project editor: Ritchey Halphen
Cover and interior design: Jonathan Norberg
Maps: Steve Jones and Johnny Molloy
Photos: Johnny Molloy, except where noted
Proofreader: Vanessa Lynn Rusch
Indexer: Meghan Miller Brawley/Potomac Indexing

 MENASHA RIDGE PRESS
An imprint of AdventureKEEN
2204 First Ave. S., Ste. 102
Birmingham, AL 35233
800-443-7227, fax 205-326-1012

Visit menasharidge.com for a complete listing of our books and for ordering information. Contact us at our website, at facebook.com/menasharidge, or at twitter.com/menasharidge with questions or comments. To find out more about who we are and what we're doing, visit blog.menasharidge.com.

Front cover: Footbridge and autumn leaves in Great Smoky Mountains National Park; photo: kurdistan/Shutterstock.
Cover inset and opposite page: Tent site at Cosby Campground (see Campground 3, page 19); photo: Chloe Kenning

5TH Edition

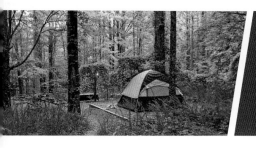

BEST TENT
Camping

Southern Appalachian and Smoky Mountains

YOUR CAR-CAMPING GUIDE TO SCENIC BEAUTY, THE SOUNDS
OF NATURE, AND AN ESCAPE FROM CIVILIZATION

Johnny Molloy

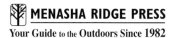

MENASHA RIDGE PRESS
Your Guide to the Outdoors Since 1982

Southern Appalachians–Smokies Campground Locator Map

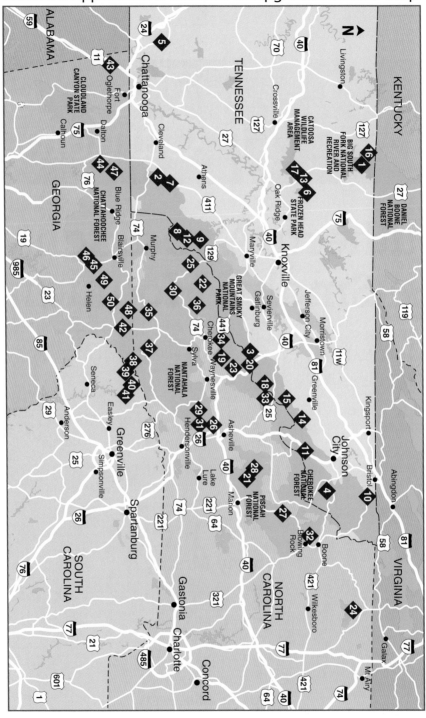

CONTENTS

TENNESSEE CAMPGROUNDS   12

NORTH CAROLINA CAMPGROUNDS   67

Map Legend

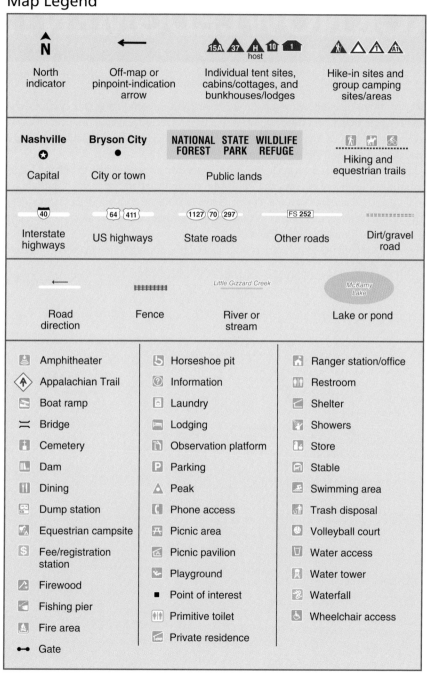

N North indicator

Off-map or pinpoint-indication arrow

Individual tent sites, cabins/cottages, and bunkhouses/lodges

Hike-in sites and group camping sites/areas

Nashville — Capital

Bryson City — City or town

NATIONAL FOREST STATE PARK WILDLIFE REFUGE — Public lands

Hiking and equestrian trails

Interstate highways

US highways

State roads

Other roads

Dirt/gravel road

Road direction

Fence

River or stream

Lake or pond

- Amphitheater
- Appalachian Trail
- Boat ramp
- Bridge
- Cemetery
- Dam
- Dining
- Dump station
- Equestrian campsite
- Fee/registration station
- Firewood
- Fishing pier
- Fire area
- Gate

- Horseshoe pit
- Information
- Laundry
- Lodging
- Observation platform
- Parking
- Peak
- Phone access
- Picnic area
- Picnic pavilion
- Playground
- Point of interest
- Primitive toilet
- Private residence

- Ranger station/office
- Restroom
- Shelter
- Showers
- Store
- Stable
- Swimming area
- Trash disposal
- Volleyball court
- Water access
- Water tower
- Waterfall
- Wheelchair access

ACKNOWLEDGMENTS

I'd like to thank the following people for their help in completing this book: Margaret Albrecht, Angie Bell, Laura Burgess, John Cox, Bryan Delay, Deal Holcomb, Steve Grayson, Tom Lauria, Bill Mai, Nancy McBee, Molly Merkle, Francisco Meyer, Michael Molloy, Tom Rogers, Karen Tate, and Deborah Turpin.

Along the way I met a lot of helpful public servants. I would like to acknowledge the contributions of personnel from the following public lands and agencies: Chattahoochee National Forest, Cherokee National Forest, Georgia State Parks, Nantahala National Forest, North Carolina State Parks, Pisgah National Forest, Sumter National Forest, South Carolina State Parks, and Tennessee State Parks.

Thanks also to all the tent campers who shared their thoughts and a cup of coffee.

—Johnny Molloy

PREFACE

Before there were cars, TVs, computers, and smartphones, life moved at a much more manageable, intimate pace. But in the age of text messages and social media, folks just can't seem to find the time to be together—and when they do, the results can be disappointing. Traditional vacations to worn-out tourist traps minimize the companionship we seek in such outings.

A tent-camping excursion is the answer to this quest for companionship. There's no dragging from attraction to attraction or fighting over where to eat. A tent-camping trip can be a time of bonding on the trail and around the fire, where experiences and sights are shared. It's a chance to experience the unique loveliness of the out-of-doors and enjoy a little fun along the way.

As we make our way through this digital age, camping allows time for introspection not found in our rush-rush world. To commune with nature is a rewarding experience for young and old alike. It is healthful for the mind and body to return to the land from which we came. Tent camping is a true vacation for all—*if* you choose the right campground.

That's where this book can help. Once you've made the commitment to go tent camping, finding the right campground can make or break your adventure. Campgrounds range in character from roadside, RV-infested "cities" to secluded hideaways nestled deep in the bosom of the mountains.

Over more than two decades, I've coursed through the Southern Appalachians and Smokies searching for the best campgrounds in the mountains of Tennessee, North Carolina, South Carolina, and Georgia. The best of the best are those nearest to a wilderness experience and not overrun by RVs. Now it's up to you to glean your favorites from this book, get back to nature, and make some memories of your own.

—J. M.

BEST
CAMPGROUNDS

BEST FOR SCENERY

BEST FOR HIKING

BEST FOR PADDLING

BEST FOR BICYCLING

BEST FOR WATERFALLS

INTRODUCTION

The Southern Appalachians. The very words give rise to images of misty, tree-topped mountains; clear whitewater streams; lush woodlands; and a biodiversity unmatched in temperate climes. At the heart of the Southern Appalachians are the Smokies, the 500,000-acre master mountain chain containing the highest, wildest country remaining in the eastern United States. The crown jewel in the chain—Great Smoky Mountains National Park, straddling Tennessee and North Carolina—justifiably attracts millions of people per year.

The allure of the national park, however, often overshadows adjacent special areas. Encircling the park are millions of acres of state-park and national-forest land that expands the range of Smoky Mountain country. This book covers not just the Smokies but also the highlands of eastern Tennessee, western North Carolina, western South Carolina, and northern Georgia.

The Southern Appalachians are a region steeped in human and natural history. These mountains played a significant role in the formation and westward expansion of our country, an expansion that oftentimes came at the expense of the Cherokee, who battled settlers and lost but eventually managed to hold on to some of their ancestral lands.

Aside from a few Civil War skirmishes, this land became a forgotten backwater, the land of "do without"—that is, until logging interests discovered its magnificent forests and began to cut them down. Thankfully, some stands were left intact; the Smokies still contain some 125,000 acres of old-growth woods. After the tree harvest in the early 1900s, the U.S. Forest Service took over the fire-scarred and eroded lands, protecting and managing the area for commercial and recreational purposes. Other special mountain places came under state protection, creating a nucleus of fine state parks.

A trip into the Southern Appalachians is sort of like a thru-hike along the Appalachian Trail. The elevation rise—from 700 to nearly 6,700 feet—creates climate zones that foster plant and animal life found from Georgia all the way to Maine. These conditions create the biodiversity that makes the Southern Appalachians special.

Generally speaking, spring takes six weeks to climb the mountains; conversely, autumn descends the mountains six weeks earlier than in the surrounding lowlands. All of this adds to the biodiversity and makes for varying weather conditions to suit your whims as you seek the wildflowers of spring, the lushness of summer, the colors of autumn, and the snows of winter. Luckily for us, we can find plenty of campgrounds tucked away in and near Smokies country.

HOW TO USE THIS GUIDEBOOK

Menasha Ridge Press welcomes you to *Best Tent Camping: Southern Appalachian and Smoky Mountains.* Whether you're new to camping or you've been sleeping in your portable shelter over decades of outdoor adventures, please review the following information. It explains how we have worked with the author to organize this book and how you can make the best use of it.

Some text on the following pages applies to all books in the Best Tent Camping series. Where this isn't the case, such as in the descriptions of weather and wildlife, the author has provided information specific to the area covered in this particular book.

THE RATING SYSTEM

As with all books in the Best Tent Camping series, the author personally experienced dozens of campgrounds and campsites to select the top 50 locations in the Southern Appalachian and Smoky Mountains. Within that universe of 50 sites, the author then ranked each one according to the six categories described below.

Each campground is superlative in its own way. For example, a site may be rated only one star in one category but perhaps five stars in another category. Our rating system allows you to choose your destination based on the attributes that are most important to you. Although these ratings are subjective, they're still excellent guidelines for finding the perfect camping experience for you and your companions.

Below and following we describe the criteria for each of the attributes in our five-star rating system:

★★★★★   The site is **ideal** in that category.

★★★★   The site is **exemplary** in that category.

★★★   The site is **very good** in that category.

★★   The site is **above average** in that category.

★   The site is **acceptable** in that category.

INDIVIDUAL RATINGS

Each campground description includes ratings for **beauty, privacy, quiet, spaciousness, security,** and **cleanliness;** each attribute is ranked from one to five stars, with five being the best. Admittedly, these ratings are subjective, but we've tried to select campgrounds that offer something for everyone.

BEAUTY

In judging beauty, I took into account what the general area has to offer as well as the campground. The most beautiful campgrounds have sites that you just don't want to leave and locations with easy access to breathtaking scenery.

PRIVACY

This rating is determined by how much your neighbors can pay attention to what you're doing, and vice versa. The best campgrounds provide plenty of green space—shrubs and trees—between adjoining sites. Such campgrounds also stagger their sites so that, for instance, the entrance to the site across the road isn't directly opposite the entrance to yours.

QUIET

My evaluations were influenced to a great extent by the presence of RVs and the kinds of visitors a park tends to get. (Campgrounds near urban areas, for example, tend to be noisy, as are those that cater to families with children.) I also considered the extent to which you could get away from the fray at a particular campground. You can expect some variation within my ratings based on whether you visit a campground during the week or on a weekend; on holiday weekends, all bets are off.

SPACIOUSNESS

This category contributes to the amount of privacy you have, but mainly it refers to how much space you have to move around in. Some sites are surprisingly large, even to the point of overkill; others are incredibly small.

SECURITY

In general, I found campgrounds in the greater Smokies to be very safe and secure, due largely to the presence of campground hosts and park rangers making the rounds. The only places where I felt security might be compromised were those remote campgrounds that saw few visitors and had no staff or rangers on duty.

CLEANLINESS

My judgments were based on the presence and remnants of past campers around the sites—trash, tent stakes, burned logs, and the like—and on the state of the restroom facilities. I did take into account that primitive toilets tend to be less tidy than modern facilities, although there seemed to me to be little reason for either to be a mess.

THE CAMPGROUND PROFILE

Each profile contains a concise but informative narrative of the campground and individual sites. In addition to the property, the recreational opportunities are also described—what's in the area and perhaps suggestions for touristy activities. This descriptive text is enhanced with three helpful sidebars: Ratings, Key Information, and Getting There (accurate driving directions that lead you to the campground from the nearest major roadway, along with GPS coordinates).

THE CAMPGROUND LOCATOR MAP AND MAP LEGEND

Use the Southern Appalachians–Smokies Campground Locator Map, opposite the Table of Contents on page iv, to assess the exact location of each campground. The campground's number appears not only on the overview map but also in the Table of Contents and on the profile's first page.

A map legend that details the symbols found on the campground-layout maps appears immediately following the Table of Contents, on page vii.

CAMPGROUND-LAYOUT MAPS

Each profile includes a detailed map of individual campsites, roads, facilities, and other key elements.

GPS CAMPGROUND-ENTRANCE COORDINATES

Readers can easily access all campgrounds in this book by using the driving directions in Getting There along with the overview maps, which show at least one major road leading into the area. But for those who enjoy using GPS technology to navigate, the book includes coordinates for each campground's entrance in latitude and longitude, expressed in degrees and decimal minutes.

To convert GPS coordinates from degrees, minutes, and seconds to the above degrees–decimal minutes format, the seconds are divided by 60. For more on GPS technology, visit usgs.gov.

A *note of caution:* A dedicated GPS unit will easily guide you to any of these campgrounds, but users of smartphone mapping apps may find that cell service is unavailable in the remote areas where a number of these hideaways are located.

WEATHER

Spring is the most variable season in this region. During March, you'll find your first signs of rebirth in the lowlands, yet trees in the high country may not be fully leafed out until June. Both winter- and summerlike weather may be experienced in spring. As summer approaches, the strong fronts weaken, and thunderstorms and haze become more frequent. Summertime rainy days can be cool, especially in the high country. In fall, continental fronts once again sweep through, clearing the air and bringing warm days and cool nights, though rain is always possible.

The first snows of winter usually arrive in November and snow can intermittently fall–April, though no permanent snowpack exists. About 20–80 inches of snow can fall during this time. Expect entire days of below-freezing weather, but be aware that temperatures can range from quite mild to bitterly cold.

FIRST AID KIT

A useful first aid kit may contain more items than you might think necessary. These are just the basics. Prepackaged kits in waterproof bags (Atwater Carey and Adventure Medical make them) are available. As a preventive measure, take along sunscreen and insect repellent. Even though quite a few items are listed here, they pack down into a small space:

- Ace bandages

- Adhesive bandages

- Antibiotic ointment (Neosporin or the generic equivalent)

- Antiseptic or disinfectant, such as Betadine or hydrogen peroxide

- Aspirin, acetaminophen (Tylenol), or ibuprofen (Advil)

- Butterfly-closure bandages

- Comb and tweezers (for removing ticks from your skin)

- Diphenhydramine (Benadryl, in case of allergic reactions)

- Epinephrine (EpiPen) in a prefilled syringe (for severe allergic reactions to outdoor mishaps such as bee stings)

- Gauze (one roll and six 4-by-4-inch compress pads)

- LED flashlight or headlamp

- Matches or lighter

- Moist towelettes

- Moleskin/Spenco 2nd Skin

- Pocketknife or multipurpose tool

- Waterproof first aid tape

- Whistle (for signaling rescuers if you get lost or injured)

WATCHWORDS FOR FLORA AND FAUNA

BEARS The Southern Appalachians and Smokies are home to black bears in abundance. Most avoid humans, but some associate humans with food and have lost their fear of people. (See page 9 for ways to bearproof your food.)

If you should have an unexpected black bear encounter, stand upright and back away slowly. Speak in a calm voice. If you spot a bear at camp or on the trail, keep your distance and make enough noise so that it's aware of your presence—*never surprise a bear.* Likewise, never get between a mother bear and her cub. Always notify campground, park, or forest staff after a bear encounter.

MOSQUITOES In the mountains, summertime is peak mosquito season, but even then these pests aren't as troublesome as they are elsewhere. At this time of year—and anytime you expect mosquitoes to be buzzing around—you may want to wear protective clothing, such as long sleeves, long pants, and socks (provided it's not too hot outside to make that impractical). Loose-fitting, light-colored clothing is best. Spray clothing with insect repellent, remembering to follow the instructions on the label and to take extra care with children.

POISON IVY, OAK, AND SUMAC Recognizing and avoiding these plants are the most effective ways to prevent the painful, itchy rashes associated with them. Poison ivy (*top right*) ranges from a thick, tree-hugging vine to a shaded ground cover, 3 leaflets to a leaf; poison oak (*center right*) occurs as either a vine or shrub, also with 3 leaflets; and poison sumac (*bottom right*) flourishes in wet wooded areas such as streambanks, with each leaf having 7–13 leaflets. Urushiol, the plants' oily sap, is responsible for the rash. Usually within 12–14 hours of exposure (but sometimes much later), raised lines and/or blisters will appear, accompanied by a terrible itch. Try not to scratch—dirty fingernails can cause an infection, and in the best case you'll spread the rash to other parts of your body.

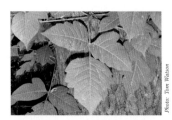

Photo: Tom Watson

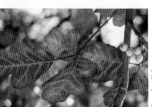

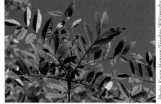

Photo: Jane Huber

Wash the rash with cold water and a mild soap or cleanser such as Tecnu, and then dry it thoroughly, applying calamine lotion or a topical cortisone cream to help soothe the itch; if the rash is painful or blistering is severe, seek medical attention. Note that any oil that gets on clothing, boots, and the like can keep spreading its misery for at least a year if you don't thoroughly clean it off, so wash everything that you think could have urushiol on it, including pets.

Photo: Kevin Hansen/Freekee/Wikimedia Commons/CC0 (creativecommons.org /license/CC0)

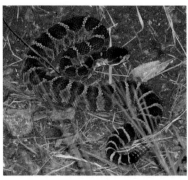

Photo: Jane Huber

SNAKES If you spend any time camping in the Southern Appalachians and Smoky Mountains, you may be surprised by the variety of snakes in the area. While most encounters will be with nonvenomous specimens, two venomous snakes do call the mountains home: the copperhead and the timber rattler. The former can be found near streams and on outcrops, whereas the latter will primarily be seen sunning on rocks. You might spend some time studying snakes before you head into the woods, but a good rule of thumb is to give *any* animal you encounter a wide berth and leave it alone.

TICKS The bane of camping trips, ticks tend to lurk in the brush, leaves, and grass that grow alongside trails. Hot summer months seem to make their numbers explode, but you should be tick-aware all year round.

Ticks, which are related to spiders, need a host to feast on in order to reproduce. The ones that alight onto you will be very small, sometimes so tiny that you won't be able to spot them until you feel the itchiness of their bite. Primarily of two varieties, deer ticks (which can carry Lyme disease) and wood ticks, both need a few hours of actual attachment before they can transmit any illness they may harbor, so the quicker you remove them the better. Ticks may settle in shoes, socks, or hats and may take several hours to actually latch on.

Wearing light-colored clothing makes ticks easier to spot; tucking the cuffs of your pants into your socks, while geeky-looking, helps keep them from latching on; and using an insect repellent with DEET helps keep them away. Visually check yourself for ticks throughout the day while you're out in the woods, and do an even more thorough check of your entire body when you're in your tent/cabin or taking a posthike shower.

If a tick should bite you, use tweezers to remove it—grab as close to the skin as possible, and firmly pull the tick loose without crushing it, making sure to remove the entire head. Then wash the area well with warm, soapy water.

Keep an eye on the bite for several days afterward to ensure that it doesn't get infected and that a rash doesn't develop. The telltale sign of Lyme infection is a bullseye-shaped rash that forms around the site of the bite; be aware, however, that you could be infected even if the rash doesn't develop. If you start experiencing flulike symptoms within a couple of weeks of getting bitten, see a doctor right away.

HAPPY CAMPING: PLANNING, ETIQUETTE, AND MORE

Few things are more disappointing than a bad camping trip—the good news is, it's really easy to have a great one. Here are a few things to consider as you prepare for your trip.

- **PLAN AHEAD.** Know your equipment, your ability, and the area where you'll be camping—and prepare accordingly. Be self-sufficient at all times; carry the necessary supplies for changes in weather or other conditions. In the same vein, reserve your site in advance when that's an option, especially if it's a weekend or holiday or if the campground is extremely popular. Also do a little research on what the campground or nearby area has to offer; campground/park staff can be extremely helpful in suggesting things to do and places to go. Finally, consider the accessibility of supplies before you go—it's a pain to have to get in the car and make a long trek in search of hot dog buns or bug spray.

- **USE CARE WHEN TRAVELING.** Stay on designated roadways. Be respectful of private property and travel restrictions. Familiarize yourself with the area you'll be traveling in by picking up a map that shows land ownership.

- **WHEN SELECTING A CAMPGROUND OR CAMPSITE, CONSIDER YOUR SPACE REQUIREMENTS.** In general, choose a single site if your group consists of 8 people or fewer, a double site for groups of up to 16 people, a triple site for groups of up to 24, or a group camping area for parties of more than 24.

- **PLAY BY THE RULES.** If you're unhappy with the site you've selected, check with the campground host for other options. Don't just grab a seemingly empty site that looks more appealing than yours—it could be reserved.

- **PICK YOUR CAMPING BUDDIES WISELY.** Make sure that everyone is on the same page regarding expectations of difficulty (amenities or the lack thereof, physical exertion, and so on), sleeping arrangements, and food requirements.

- **DRESS FOR THE SEASON.** Educate yourself on the temperature highs and lows of the specific part of the state you plan to visit. It may be warm at night in the summer in your backyard, but up in the mountains it will often be quite chilly.

- **PITCH YOUR TENT ON A LEVEL SURFACE,** either on a tent pad at the camp-site or a surface covered with leaves, pine straw, or grass. Use a tarp or specially designed footprint to thwart ground moisture and to protect the tent floor. Before you pitch, do some site cleanup, such as picking up small rocks and sticks that can damage your tent floor and make sleep uncomfortable. If you have a separate rainfly but aren't sure you'll need it, keep it rolled up at the base of your tent in case it starts raining late at night.

- **PACK A SLEEPING PAD IF LYING ON THE GROUND MAKES YOU UNCOMFORTABLE.** Pads in a wide range of sizes and thicknesses are sold at outdoor stores. Inflatable pads are also available—don't try to improvise with a home air mattress, which conducts heat away from the body and tends to deflate as you sleep.

- **DON'T HANG OR TIE CLOTHESLINES, HAMMOCKS, AND EQUIPMENT ON OR TO TREES.** Even if you see other campers doing this, be responsible and do your part to reduce damage to trees and shrubs.

- **IF YOU TEND TO USE THE BATHROOM FREQUENTLY AT NIGHT, PLAN AHEAD.** Leaving a comfy sleeping bag and stumbling around in the dark to find a place to heed nature's call—be it a vault toilet, a full restroom, or just the woods—is no fun. Keep a flashlight and any other accoutrements you may need within easy reach, and know exactly where to head in the dark.

- **LIKEWISE, KNOW HOW TO GO IN THE BACKCOUNTRY.** If you're camping at a primitive site, bringing large jugs of water and a portable toilet is the easiest and most environmentally friendly solution. A variety of portable toilets are available from outdoors suppliers; in a pinch, a 5-gallon bucket fitted with a toilet seat and lined with a heavy-duty plastic trash bag will work just as well. (Don't forget to pack out the bag.) A second, less desirable method is to dig an 8-inch-deep cathole. It should be located at least 200 yards from campsites, trails, and water, in an inconspicuous location with as much undergrowth as possible. Cover the hole with a thin layer of soil after each use, and *don't burn or bury your toilet paper*—pack it out in resealable plastic bags. If you plan to stay at the campsite for several days, dig a new hole each day, being careful to replace the topsoil over the hole from the day before. In addition to the plastic bags, your outdoor-toilet cache should include a garden trowel, toilet paper, and wet wipes. Select a trowel with a well-designed handle that can also double as a toilet paper dispenser.

- **IF YOU'RE CAMPING AT A DEVELOPED SITE, DON'T SKIMP ON FOOD.** Plan tasty meals, and bring everything you'll need to prep, cook, eat, and clean up. That said, don't duplicate equipment such as cooking pots among the members of your group.

- **KEEP A CLEAN COOKING AREA,** and pick up food scraps on the ground both during and after your visit. Maintain a group trash bag, and be sure to secure it in your vehicle at night. Many campgrounds have a pack-in/pack-out rule, and that means everything: no cheating by tossing orange peels, eggshells, or apple cores in the shrubs.

- **DO YOUR PART TO PREVENT BEARS FROM BECOMING CONDITIONED TO SEEKING HUMAN FOOD.** In the Southern Appalachians and Smokies, where bears abound, this is especially important. The constant search for food influences every aspect of a bear's life, so when camping in bear country, store food in your vehicle or in bearproof containers. Keep food (including canned goods, soft drinks, and beer) and garbage secured, and don't take food with you into your tent. You'll also need to stow scented or flavored toiletries such as deodorant, toothpaste, and lip balm, as well as cooking grease and pet food. Common sense and adherence to the simple rules posted in the campgrounds will help keep you and the bears safe and healthy. (See page 5 for what to do if you encounter a bear.)

- **USE ESTABLISHED FIRE RINGS, AND BE AWARE OF FIRE RESTRICTIONS.** Make sure that your fire is totally extinguished whenever you leave the area. If you cook with a Dutch oven, use a fire pan and elevate it to avoid scorching or burning the ground. Don't burn garbage in your campfire—trash fires smell awful and often don't burn completely, plus fire rings fill with burned litter over time. Also check ahead to see if bringing your own firewood is allowed. If it's not, buying firewood on-site (if available) may be preferable to gathering deadfall, which is frequently green and/or wet.

- **DON'T WASH DISHES AND LAUNDRY OR BATHE IN STREAMS AND LAKES.** Food scraps are unsightly and can be potentially harmful to fish, and even biodegradable soaps can be harmful to fragile aquatic environments.

- **BE A GOOD NEIGHBOR.** Observe quiet hours, keep noise to a minimum, and keep your pets leashed and under control.

- **MOST IMPORTANT, LEAVE YOUR CAMP CLEANER THAN YOU FOUND IT.** Pick up all trash and microlitter in your site, including in your fire ring. Disperse leftover brush used for firewood.

VENTURING AWAY FROM THE CAMPGROUND

If you decide to go for a hike, bike, or other excursion into the boondocks, here are some safety tips.

- **LET SOMEONE AT HOME OR AT CAMP KNOW WHERE YOU'LL BE GOING AND HOW LONG YOU EXPECT TO BE GONE.** Also let him or her know when you return.

- **SIGN IN AND OUT OF ANY TRAIL REGISTERS PROVIDED.** Leave notes on trail conditions if space allows—that's your opportunity to alert others to any problems you encounter.

- **DON'T ASSUME THAT YOUR PHONE WILL WORK ON THE TRAIL.** Reception may be spotty or nonexistent, especially on a trail embraced by towering trees.

- **ALWAYS CARRY FOOD AND WATER, EVEN FOR A SHORT HIKE.** And bring more water than you think you'll need. Boil, filter, or chemically treat water from a stream before drinking it.

- **ASK QUESTIONS.** Public-land employees are on hand to help.

- **STAY ON DESIGNATED TRAILS.** If you become disoriented, assess your current direction, and then retrace your steps to the point where you went astray. Using a map, compass, and/or GPS unit, and keeping in mind what you've passed thus far, reorient yourself and trust your judgment on which way to continue. If you become absolutely unsure of how to continue, return to your vehicle the way you came in. Should you become completely lost, staying put and waiting for help is most often the best option for adults and always the best option for children.

Paddling Fontana Lake (see Tsali Campground, campground 36, page 119)

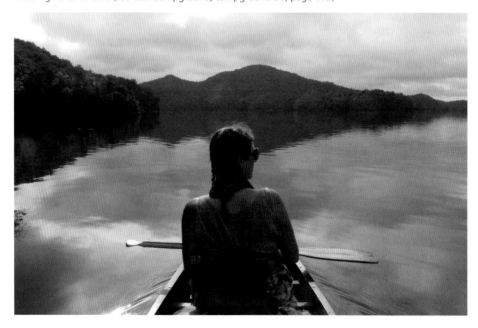

- **CARRY A WHISTLE.** It could save your life if you get lost or hurt.

- **BE ESPECIALLY CAREFUL WHEN CROSSING STREAMS.** Whether you're fording a stream or crossing on a log, make every step count. If you have any doubt about maintaining your balance on a log, ford the stream instead: use a trekking pole or stout stick for balance and *face upstream as you cross.* If a stream seems too deep to ford, turn back.

- **BE CAREFUL AT OVERLOOKS.** While these areas provide spectacular views, they're also potentially hazardous. Stay back from the edge of outcrops, and be absolutely sure of your footing.

- **STANDING DEAD TREES AND DAMAGED LIVING TREES POSE A SIGNIFICANT HAZARD TO HIKERS.** These trees may have loose or broken limbs that could fall at any time. While walking beneath trees, and when choosing a spot to rest or enjoy a snack, *look up.*

- **KNOW THE SYMPTOMS OF SUBNORMAL BODY TEMPERATURE, OR HYPOTHERMIA.** Shivering and forgetfulness are the two most common indicators. Hypothermia can occur at any elevation, even in the summer—especially if you're wearing lightweight cotton clothing. If symptoms develop, get to shelter, hot liquids, and dry clothes as soon as possible.

- **LIKEWISE, KNOW THE SYMPTOMS OF ABNORMALLY HIGH BODY TEMPERATURE, OR HYPERTHERMIA.** Lightheadedness and weakness are the first two indicators. If you feel these symptoms, find some shade, drink some water, remove as many layers of clothing as practical, and stay put until you cool down. Marching through heat exhaustion leads to heatstroke—which can be fatal. If you should be sweating and you're not, that's the signature warning sign. If you or a hiking partner is experiencing heatstroke, do whatever you can to get cool and find help.

- **MOST IMPORTANT, TAKE ALONG YOUR BRAIN.** Think before you act. Watch your step. Plan ahead.

TENNESSEE CAMPGROUNDS

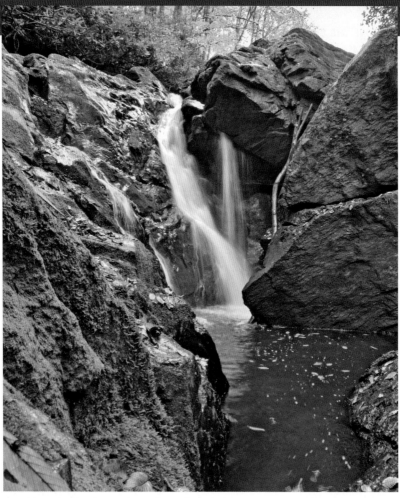

Upper Laurel Fork Falls is within walking distance of Dennis Cove Campground (page 22).

Bandy Creek Campground

Beauty: ★★★ Privacy: ★★★ Spaciousness: ★★★★ Quiet: ★★★ Security: ★★★★ Cleanliness: ★★★★★

Bandy Creek Campground lies at the heart of the 100,000-acre Big South Fork National River and Recreation Area.

The National Park Service is catching on. It realizes there are two divergent groups that use campgrounds: tent campers and RVers. Here at Bandy Creek Campground, the park service has designated a tent-only loop. This is a good thing, because having a recommended campground in the Big South Fork completes the outdoor package.

Protected since 1974, the Big South Fork features wild rivers, steep gorges, thick forests, and remnants of human history atop the Cumberland Plateau. A well-developed trail system with paths leaving directly from the campground makes exploring the Big South Fork easy. There are also mountain biking, paddling, fishing, and rafting opportunities.

Bandy Creek Campground is a large complex with a total of four camping loops. A recreational area and the park's visitor center are nearby. Loop A is the only loop reserved exclusively for tent campers. It is separated from the rest of the campground, being off to the left after you pass the campground registration booth. My most recent stay was in A, at campsite 14. Most of the camping area is wooded. A few sites back up to a field and the recreation complex, which includes a swimming pool and a playground for young campers. Since Bandy Creek is atop the plateau, the forest is mixed hardwood with oaks, tulip trees,

A hiker visits the John Litton Farm.

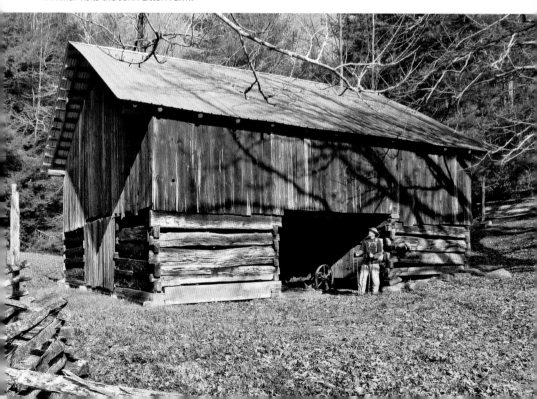

KEY INFORMATION

CONTACT: 423-286-8368, nps.gov/biso; reservations: 877-444-6777, recreation.gov

OPEN: April 1–October 31; limited sites open year-round

SITES: 181 (49 nonelectric, 96 electric, 35 group sites)

EACH SITE HAS: Tent pad, fire grate, picnic table, lantern post

WHEELCHAIR ACCESS: 8 sites

ASSIGNMENT: First-come, first-served and by reservation

REGISTRATION: At campground entrance station or self-register on-site

FACILITIES: Piped water, flush toilets, hot showers

PARKING: At campsites only, 2 vehicles/site

FEES: $20/night nonelectric sites, $25–$32/night electric sites, $125/night group sites

ELEVATION: 1,500'

RESTRICTIONS:

PETS: On leash 6' or shorter

QUIET HOURS: 10 p.m.–6 a.m.

FIRES: In fire grates only

ALCOHOL: At campsites only

VEHICLES: 70' length limit

OTHER: 6 people/site; 14-day stay limit; food must be stored in vehicle or trailer unless you're eating it

---

and Virginia pine. The campsites themselves are mostly open, bordered by dense woodland. A miniloop extends from Loop A and contains four out-of-the-way sites. Beyond the first miniloop, campsites with paved parking areas extend on either side of the road as it rises slightly, passing one of the two most complete washhouses I've ever encountered. The buildings are designed to complement the local architecture and have a water fountain, piped water, flush toilets, showers, and even a two-basin sink for washing dishes.

Farther on, the road divides and arrives at one of the two bad sites in the campground: site 32 is adjacent to the water tower, while site 2 backs up to the swimming pool. As Loop A swings around, there is a miniloop off of it. This loop contains seven wooded sites that are the most private in the campground. The main road passes the second washhouse. Three other water pumps are dispersed among the 49 well-kept sites. The rest of the campground contains 96 sites. Only Loop D, with 52 sites, is open during the winter, for tents and RVs. The pool is open from June to Labor Day, but the rest of this park is ready to be explored year-round.

Hiking is very popular. And why not? Trails lace the immediate area. The John Litton–General Slavens Loop traverses 6 miles of surrounding countryside. It descends to the valley where the John Litton Farm stands, passes a large rock house, and climbs back up to the campground via Fall Branch Falls. If you prefer a trail with more human and natural history, take the Oscar Blevins Loop. It is a moderate, 3.6-mile loop that passes the Blevins Farm, some large trees, and more of the steep bluffs that characterize the Cumberland Plateau. Another hiking option is the easy Bandy Creek Campground Loop. It is a short, 1.3-mile family hike that offers a good introduction to the area. Want more trails? Stop by the visitor center, and they can point you in the right direction. If you don't feel like walking, ride a horse. The nearby Bandy Creek Stables offer guided rides for a fee. Water enthusiasts should drive the short distance to Leatherwood Ford and the Big South Fork for aquatic recreation. There the river flows through a scenic gorge with steep cliffs soaring to the sky. Exciting rapids and decent fishing can be found both upstream and down. Check the visitor center for river conditions. Mountain biking is growing in popularity too. Obviously you won't be spending much time relaxing at the campground. There is simply too much to see and do. Come see the Big South Fork and you will have spent your time well.

Bandy Creek Campground

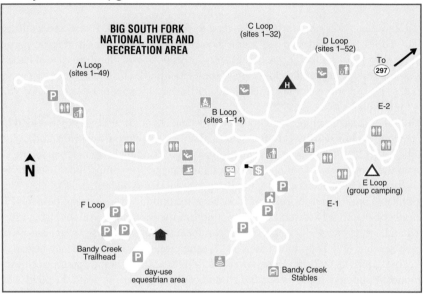

GETTING THERE

From I-75, take Exit 141 (Oneida/Huntsville). Turn onto TN 63 West, and drive 4.4 miles. Keep left to continue onto TN 297 West, and drive 15.8 miles. Turn right onto US 27 North, and drive 5.4 miles. Turn left onto Verdun Road, and drive 0.8 mile. Turn right and then immediately left to continue on Verdun Road; then drive another 0.6 mile. Turn left onto TN 297 West, and drive 7.2 miles. Turn right at the sign for Bandy Creek Campground.

GPS COORDINATES N36° 29.259' W84° 41.440'

Chilhowee Campground

Beauty: ★★★★ Privacy: ★★★ Spaciousness: ★★★★ Quiet: ★★★ Security: ★★★★★ Cleanliness: ★★★★★

This mountaintop campground offers plenty to keep campers busy and happy.

The Chilhowee experience starts on the road to the campground. Forest Service Road 77 is a U.S. Forest Service–designated scenic byway that climbs 7 miles to the campground. Don't rush the trip—pull off at one of the cleared overlooks, and enjoy the view of Parksville Lake below and the mountains and valleys undulating in the distance. Once you've made the pull to the top and seen the campground, it's the nearby activities that will keep you up there for a while.

This mountaintop campground is a cool retreat on hot summer days. Popular with families, many of whom return year after year, Chilhowee fills up on weekends and holidays. Although there are 25 sites with electric hookups, tent camping is the norm here; the steep drive up the mountain discourages most RVs and trailers. The campground itself is spread across three distinct areas. Loops A and B are the oldest and highest, built in the 1930s by the Civilian Conservation Corps, but have been retrofitted with electrical hookups. They are nestled beneath a hardwood forest in a dip on the mountain. Water spigots are well placed and accessible to all campers. Two comfort stations with flush toilets are available for each sex, but only Loop B has showers. A campground host keeps the area clean, safe, and secure. Loops C, D, E, and F are newer and more spacious. They are placed according to the mountainous terrain and have more ground cover for privacy beneath the piney woods. Two comfort stations serve the four loops, but only Loop F has showers. Loop E has electrical hookups. Water is easily accessible in these loops.

The third area, for overflow camping, is in an open, grassy field ringed by woods. It has one comfort station, but no shower, for the 23 overflow sites. There is one water source

A scenic trail heads southeast from the campground to Benton Falls.

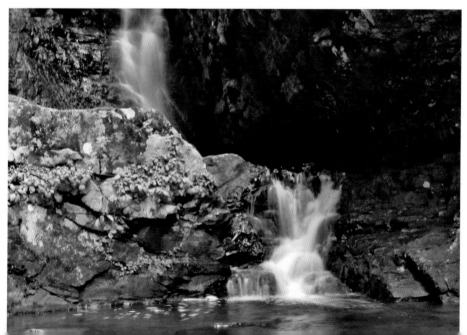

CONTACT: 423-338-3300, www.fs.usda.gov
/cherokee; reservations: 877-444-6777,
recreation.gov

OPEN: April–November; limited sites open
year-round

SITES: 61

EACH SITE HAS: Picnic table, grill,
lantern post

WHEELCHAIR ACCESS: Some sites

ASSIGNMENT: First-come, first-served and
by reservation

REGISTRATION: Self-register on-site

FACILITIES: Flush toilets, warm showers,
drinking water

PARKING: At campsites and walk-in parking
area only

FEES: $12/night nonelectric sites, $15–$20/
night electric sites

ELEVATION: 2,600'

RESTRICTIONS:
PETS: On leash only

QUIET HOURS: 10 p.m.–6 a.m.

FIRES: In fire grates only

ALCOHOL: Prohibited

VEHICLES: No overnight parking in
day-use lot

OTHER: Maximum 5 people/site; 14-day
stay limit

here. Too close together, the sites are neither spacious nor private, but campers make the most of it because of the numerous recreational opportunities nearby.

Want to take a hike? You won't have to go far from camp. The Azalea Trail begins in Loop F, climbing the ridge above the campground then making a 2-mile loop back. Or keep going on the Clear Creek Trail to the northern rim of the Rock Creek Gorge Scenic Area. Benton Falls Trail starts near McKamy Lake and travels 1.6 miles to end at the 65-foot falls. Be careful: it gets steep at the very end. Bicyclists can stretch their legs too. Pedal the Red Leaf Trail to Benton Falls or ride the Arbutus Trail or additional mountain biking trails.

If all that exercise gets you steamed up, take a dip in 3-acre McKamy Lake. At the swimming beach on the northern end, sunbathers lie in the sun then cool off in the water. Anglers may try to catch bream and bass from the shore or toss a line from a small nonmotorized boat. Visible from the mountain along US 64 is the famed Ocoee River. For years, the water was diverted from the streambed into an old wooden flume to generate power. When the flume began to leak, the water was again let loose into the Ocoee riverbed. Paddling enthusiasts realized that the long-lost rapids would be a wonderful challenge in a canoe, kayak, or raft, and the new recreational opportunity has been an economic boon to the area ever since, with paddlers coming from all over the world to test the waters. A bevy of outfitters will guide you down the crashing whitewater on a hair-raising raft ride.

GETTING THERE

From I-75 near Cleveland, take Exit 25 (Cleveland/Dayton). Turn onto TN 60 South, and drive about 4.2 miles; then use the right lane to merge onto US 64 East (Ocoee). Drive 15.1 miles; then turn left onto Oswald Road/Forest Service Road 77 (just past the Ocoee District Ranger Station). Drive about 7.3 miles; Chilhowee Campground will be on your right.

GPS COORDINATES N35° 09.004' W84° 36.267'

Chilhowee Campground: Loops A & B

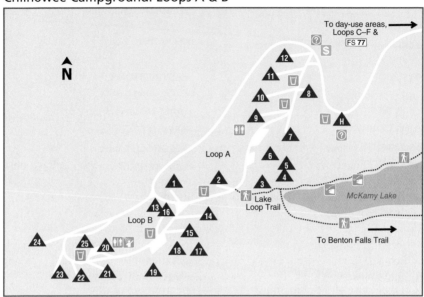

Chilhowee Campground: Loops C–F

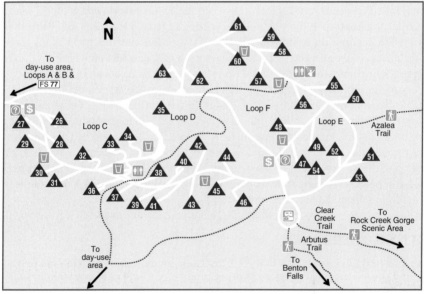

⛺ Cosby Campground

Beauty: ★★★★★ Privacy: ★★★ Spaciousness: ★★★★ Quiet: ★★★★ Security: ★★★★ Cleanliness: ★★★★★

Located off the principal Smokies tourist circuit, this cool, wooded campground makes an ideal base for exploring the virgin forests and high country of the Cosby–Greenbrier area.

Set on a slight incline in what once was pioneer farmland, this attractive terraced campground is surrounded on three sides by mountains. The large camping area is situated between the confluence of Rock and Cosby Creeks. On my trips to the area I have rarely seen Cosby Campground crowded, whereas other equally large Smokies campgrounds are sometimes cramped, noisy, and overflowing. Several loops expand the campground, and bathrooms are conveniently located throughout the site.

Now beautifully reforested, this area is rich in Smoky Mountain history. Cosby was one of the most heavily settled areas in the Smokies before Uncle Sam began buying up land for a national park in the East. The farmland was marginal anyway, so, in order to supplement their income, Cosby residents set up moonshine stills in the remote hollows of this rugged country. As a result, Cosby became known as the "moonshine capital of the world."

In remote brush-choked hollows along little streamlets, "blockaders"—as moonshiners were known—established stills. Before too long they had clear whiskey, or "mountain dew," ready for consumption. Government agents known as revenuers, who were determined to stop the production and sale of "corn likker," battled the moonshiners throughout the hills.

You can hike to Mount Cammerer via Low Gap from Cosby Campground.

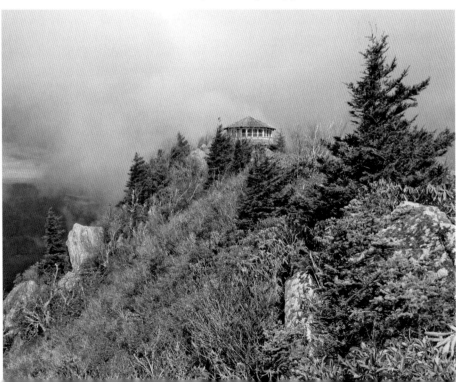

KEY INFORMATION

CONTACT: 865-436-1200, nps.gov/grsm;
reservations: 877-444-6777, recreation.gov

OPEN: Loop A, late March–October;
Loop B, late May–October

SITES: 157

EACH SITE HAS: Picnic table, fire pit,
lantern post

ASSIGNMENT: First-come, first-served or by
reservation (26 sites)

WHEELCHAIR ACCESS: Some sites

REGISTRATION: At campground entrance hut

AMENITIES: Water, flush toilets

PARKING: At campsites only, 2 vehicles/site

FEE: $17.50/night

ELEVATION: 2,459'

RESTRICTIONS:

PETS: On leash only

QUIET HOURS: 10 p.m.–6 a.m.

FIRES: In fire pits only

ALCOHOL: At campsites only

VEHICLES: 25' length limit

OTHER: 6 people/site; 14-day stay limit

It is doubtful that any stills operate within the park boundaries today; however, in other areas of Cocke County, someone is surely practicing the art of "feeding the furnace, stirring the mash, and judging the bead."

Its past is what makes Cosby so interesting. Trails split off in every direction, allowing campers to explore the human and natural history of this area. Follow the Lower Mount Cammerer Trail 1.5 mile to Sutton Ridge Overlook. On the way to the overlook, watch for signs of homesteaders from bygone days: rock walls, springs, and old chimneys. At the overlook you'll get a good lay of the land: Gabes Mountain to your east, the main crest of the Smokies to your south, the Cosby Valley below, and the hills of East Tennessee on the horizon.

Another hiking option is the Gabes Mountain Trail. Along its 6.6-mile length, this trail passes picturesque Hen Wallow Falls and meanders through huge old-growth hemlock and tulip trees and scattered old homesites. Turn around at the Sugar Cove backcountry campsite.

Don't forget to explore nearby Greenbrier. The 4-mile Ramsay Cascades Trail traverses virgin forest and ends at a picturesque waterfall that showers hikers with a fine mist. The Brushy Mountain Trail winds its way through several vegetation zones to an impressive view of the looming mass of Mount LeConte above and Gatlinburg below. Grapeyard Ridge Trail is the area's most historical and secluded hike. Walk old country paths along Rhododendron Creek and count the homesites amid fields slowly being obscured by the forest. At 3 miles, just before the Injun Creek backcountry campsite, look for the old tractor that made its last turn in these Smoky Mountains.

The crown jewel trek from Cosby Campground is the 6-mile hike to the restored Mount Cammerer fire tower. Built on a rock outcrop, it was formerly called White Rock by Tennesseans and Sharp Top by Carolinians. It has since been renamed Mount Cammerer, after Arno B. Cammerer, the former director of the National Park Service. Restored by a philanthropic outfit called Friends of the Smokies, the squat, wood-and-stone tower was originally built by the Civilian Conservation Corps during the Depression. The 360° view is well worth the climb. To the north is the Cosby Valley and the rock cut of I-40. Mount Sterling and its fire tower are to the south. The main crest of the Smokies stands to the west, and a wave of mountains fades away on the eastern horizon.

Cosby Campground is a real winner. Where else can you set up your tent in the middle of history? In the summer, naturalist programs in the campground amphitheater offer campers a chance to learn more about the area from rangers and other park personnel. The campground's size allows campers to set up near or away from others to achieve their perfect degree of solitude. If you are in the mood for company, however, the tourist mecca of Gatlinburg is nearby. There, you can visit an Elvis museum, see a musical revue, stock up on souvenirs, and stuff yourself with taffy—and even get some locally made legal moonshine.

Cosby Campground

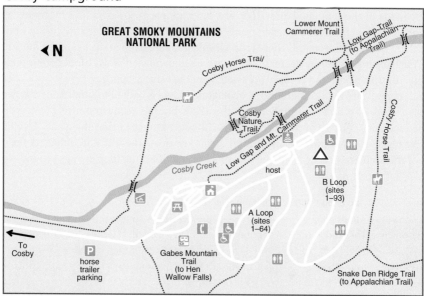

GETTING THERE

From Gatlinburg, take US 321 North for 18.1 miles, until it comes to a T-intersection with TN 32. Turn right onto TN 32 South, and drive 1.2 miles; then turn right into the signed Cosby section of Great Smoky Mountains National Park. Drive 2.1 miles to the campground registration hut.

From I-40, take Exit 447 (Hartford Road). From westbound I-40, turn left onto Big Creek Road and then immediately right onto Hartford Road, or, from eastbound I-40, turn right onto Hartford Road. Drive about 2.1 miles; then turn left onto Lindsey Gap Road, and drive 1.3 miles. Turn left onto Ground Hog Road, and drive 1.2 miles; then turn right onto TN 32 North, and drive 1.6 miles. Turn left into the signed Cosby section of Great Smoky Mountains National Park, and drive 2.1 miles to the campground registration hut.

GPS COORDINATES N35° 45.300' W83° 12.474'

4

Dennis Cove Campground

Beauty: ★★★★ Privacy: ★★★ Spaciousness: ★★★★ Quiet: ★★★★ Security: ★★★ Cleanliness: ★★★

Recreational opportunities abound at every turn.

Camp here to enjoy the delightful national forest that surrounds this fine campground. It can be busy on weekends, but no busier than other national forest campgrounds. Fishing and hiking opportunities at Dennis Cove will help you recoup some of the investment you've made in these public lands. They are, after all, yours to enjoy. The intimate campground is set in a small flat alongside Laurel Fork. A steep, sloped ridge and thickly wooded creek hem in the campground. There is no mistake, you are deep in the bosom of the Southern Appalachians. The Appalachian Trail, with its unparalleled views of Eastern mountain beauty, runs near here and is easily accessed from the campground.

As you pull into the campground, a small grassy glade is bathed in sunlight in this deeply forested cove. This area was timbered in the 1920s but has recovered nicely. A teardrop-shaped loop contains 12 of the 15 campsites. The first two sites abut the glade. Two other sites lie inside the loop, which has a grassy area of its own. The next three sites on the outside of the loop are heavily shaded by hemlock trees. Then the loop swings around to the

Dennis Cove Falls lies a short distance from the campground.

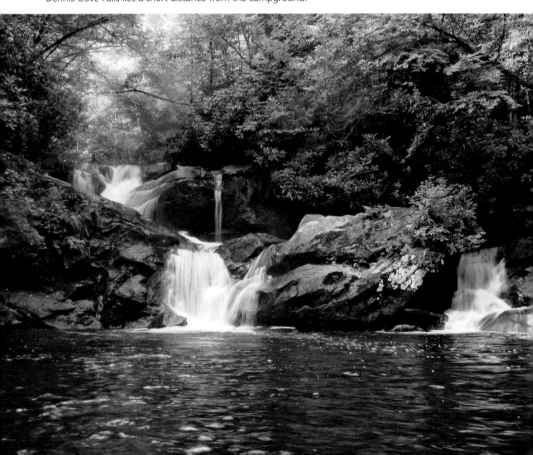

KEY INFORMATION

CONTACT: 423-735-1500, www.fs.usda.gov
/cherokee; reservations: 877-444-6777,
recreation.gov

OPEN: Late-April–mid-October

SITES: 15

EACH SITE HAS: Tent pad, fire ring,
lantern post, picnic table

ASSIGNMENT: First-come, first-served and
by reservation

WHEELCHAIR ACCESS: Yes, 2 campsites

REGISTRATION: Self-register on-site

AMENITIES: Water spigot, flush toilets

PARKING: At campsites only

FEE: $10/night

ELEVATION: 2,650'

RESTRICTIONS:

PETS: On leash 6' or shorter

QUIET HOURS: 10 p.m.–6 a.m.

FIRES: In fire rings only

ALCOHOL: Prohibited

VEHICLES: None

OTHER: 14-day stay limit

four most popular sites, situated alongside gurgling Laurel Fork. The understory is denser here, owing to the abundance of rhododendron, which thrives in the cool, moist environs of Appalachian streams. Two more sites are widely spaced on the outside of the gravel road as it completes the loop. Hardwoods mix with a few white pines in these flat sites.

There are three other sites on the other side of the gravel road leading to the loop. These sites, large by any campground's standard, are carved out of the steep hill bordering Dennis Cove. Each site is separated by woodland from the others. If it has rained lately, as it often does here, these spots are your best bet for a dry campsite.

Three water spigots are evenly dispersed about the loop. Just turn the handle and the water is yours. A small comfort station, with one flush toilet for each sex, is 100 feet off the loop away from the campground entrance. Moss growing on the stones in this area is evidence that the campground has been around a long time; however, it is revamped periodically. A campground host keeps things safe and clean during the warm season.

Explore your surroundings after you've set up camp. The waterfall enthusiast has three destinations within walking distance. Walk the half mile back toward Hampton and you'll soon see a creek on the left. Follow the old 0.8-mile trail, often trod by Dennis Cove campers, up to Coon Den Falls. If you continue beyond the falls, you can access the Appalachian Trail (AT). Turn left and climb along White Rocks Mountain to Moreland Gap trail shelter. A little farther back down Forest Service Road 50 toward Hampton you'll find more of the AT. Leave directly from Forest Service Road 50 and follow the old railroad grade into the Laurel Fork Gorge and the Pond Mountain Wilderness. Rock outcrops and a riverine environment characterize the path to Laurel Falls. If you keep going, you'll end up in Maine.

Forest Trail 39 leaves from the campground and follows Laurel Fork into the high country. This trail crosses Laurel Fork several times as it leads upstream to Upper Laurel Falls. The trail is popular with anglers, who match wits with the secretive brown trout that inhabit Laurel Fork. The Lacy Trap Trail, which leaves Laurel Fork in a field, leads to the AT and offers a great loop hike that I have enjoyed. The recreational opportunities available near Dennis Cove are limited only by your desire. The 6,000-acre Pond Mountain Wilderness is close by, as is mountain-rimmed Watauga Lake. So find some time and head on over.

Dennis Cove Campground

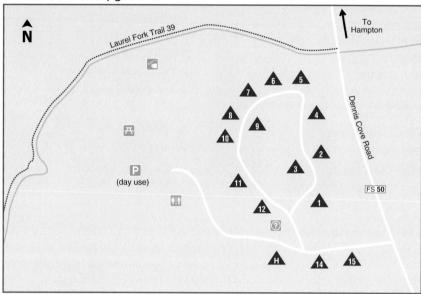

GETTING THERE

From I-26 near Johnson City, take Exit 24 (TN 67/US 321/Elizabethton), and merge onto TN 67 East/US 321 North. Drive 5 miles; then turn right onto TN 362 North, and drive 5.7 miles. Continue straight onto TN 361 East, and drive 2.4 miles. Turn left onto US 19E North, and drive 2.0 miles into Hampton. Turn right onto US 321 South, and drive 0.8 mile. Turn right onto Dennis Cove Road, and drive 4.9 twisting, turning miles. Dennis Cove Campground will be on your right.

GPS COORDINATES N36° 15.432' W82° 06.612'

5

Foster Falls Campground

Beauty: ★★★ Privacy: ★★★ Spaciousness: ★★★★★ Quiet: ★★★ Security: ★★★★★ Cleanliness: ★★★★

Foster Falls Campground can be your headquarters for exploring the South Cumberland Recreation Area.

The south end of the Cumberland Plateau has some of the wildest, roughest country in Tennessee. Sheer bluffs border deep gulfs—what natives call gorges. In these gorges flow wild streams strewn with rock gardens hosting a variety of vegetation. Intermingled within this is a human history of logging and mining that has given way to the nonextractive use of nature: ecotourism.

Foster Falls Campground has been taken over by South Cumberland State Park. It offers a safe and appealing base for your camping experience in the South Cumberlands. The campground is situated on a level, wooded tract near the state park's Foster Falls trailhead. It features the classic loop design, only the loop is so large it seems to engulf the 26 sites spread along it. Hardwoods give way to pines as you head toward the forested back of the loop. An interesting tree in the campground is the umbrella magnolia. Its leaves can reach two feet in length, causing its limbs to sag during the summer. Look for the tree along the campground entrance road and among sites 1–10.

View along the Fiery Gizzard Trail

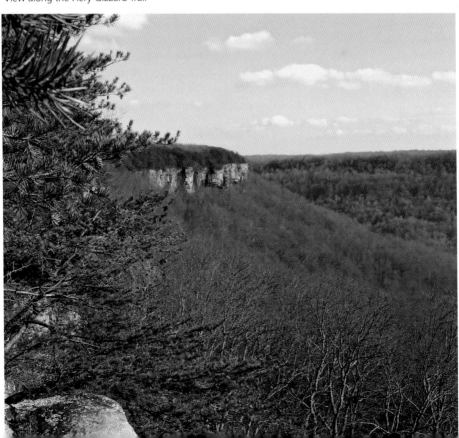

KEY INFORMATION

CONTACT: 931-924-2980, tnstateparks.com

OPEN: Year-round

SITES: 26

EACH SITE HAS: Fire grate, picnic table, lantern post

WHEELCHAIR ACCESS: Yes, 1 campsite

ASSIGNMENT: Reservations required

REGISTRATION: Resident manager will come by to register you

AMENITIES: Water spigots, hot showers, flush toilets

PARKING: At campsites or lot

FEES: $18/night plus $5 reservation fee

ELEVATION: 1,750'

RESTRICTIONS:

PETS: On leash 6' or shorter

QUIET HOURS: 9 p.m.–sunrise

FIRES: In fire grates only

ALCOHOL: Not allowed

VEHICLES: None

OTHER: 14-day stay

The spindly, second-growth tree trunks form a light understory, but the campsites are so diffused that site privacy isn't compromised. The understory actually lends a parklike atmosphere to the campground.

Foster Falls has some of the most spacious campsites I've ever seen. The large concrete picnic tables have concrete bases to keep your feet clean during those rainy times. Tent pads are conspicuously absent, but there is plenty of flat terrain for pitching your tent.

Water spigots are handy to all campsites. The state park has renovated the bathhouse, adding hot showers since taking over the campground. Quite often, your camping companions will be rock climbers, for Foster Falls has quietly emerged as the premier rock-climbing area in the Southeast.

South Cumberland State Park has nine different units, totaling more than 25,000 acres, ready for you to enjoy. For starters, a connector trail leaves the campground to Foster Falls. Here, you can take the short loop trail that leads to the base of 120-foot Foster Falls or intersect the south end of the Fiery Gizzard Trail and see Foster Falls from the top looking down. If you take the Fiery Gizzard Trail, you will be rewarded with views into Little Gizzard and Fiery Gizzard gulfs. Trail signs point out the rock bluffs where rock climbers ply their trade. The first 2.5 miles offer many vistas and small waterfalls where side creeks plunge into the gorge below. My favorite view is from the Laurel Creek Gorge Overlook, where rock bluffs on the left meld into forested drop-offs beyond, contrasting with the flat plateau in the background.

Other must-sees in the South Cumberlands are Grundy Forest, Grundy Lakes, Savage Gulf, and the Great Stone Door. Download a map and explore all the sights. Grundy Forest contains about 4 miles of the most feature-packed hiking you can ask for: four major waterfalls, swimming holes, rockhouses, old trees, old mines, and strange rock formations. Just remember to watch where you walk, as the trails can be rough.

Grundy Lakes State Park is on the National Historic Register. Once the site of mining activity, this area has seen prison labor, revolts, and the cooling down of the infamous Lone Rock coke ovens. The Lone Rock Trail will lead you to all the interesting sites.

At Savage Gulf State Natural Area, three gorges converge to form a giant crow's foot. An extensive trail system connects the cliffs, waterfalls, sinkholes, and historic sites of the area.

The Great Stone Door is a 10- by 100-foot crack in the Big Creek Gorge that was used by Indians who traversed Savage Gulf.

The campground at Foster Falls is pleasant enough to warrant a stay of a week or more, and that's about how long you'll need to get a good taste of the South Cumberland Recreation Area.

Foster Falls Campground

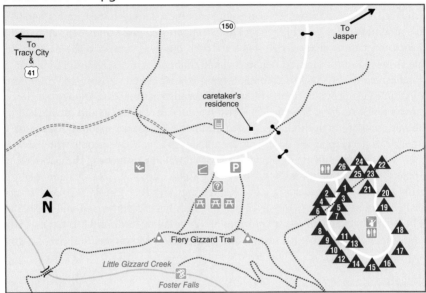

GETTING THERE

From I-24 west of Chattanooga, take Exit 155 (TN 28/Jasper/Dunlap). Turn onto TN 28 North, and drive 1.5 miles. Use the right lane to take the US 41/US 64/US 72 ramp to Jasper. Turn left onto US 41 North, and drive 0.8 mile into Jasper. Turn right to stay on US 41 North, and drive 1.2 miles. Turn left to stay on US 41 North, and drive 7.5 miles. Turn left at the sign for Foster Falls, and then drive 0.3 miles to the campground, on your left.

GPS COORDINATES N35° 10.940' W85° 40.312'

6

Frozen Head State Park Campground

Beauty: ★★★★★ Privacy: ★★★ Spaciousness: ★★★★ Quiet: ★★★★★ Security: ★★★★★ Cleanliness: ★★★★★

Stay at Frozen Head and explore the waterfalls, rock shelters, and mountaintop caprocks of the Cumberland Mountains.

Frozen Head is a lesser-known jewel of a state park tucked away in the Cumberland Mountains, a mountain range west of the Smokies. Steep forested peaks and deep valleys diffused with rock formations characterize this state park that was settled in the early 1800s by simple farmers. But the land, so rich in coal and timber resources, was sold to the state for the establishment of the now-infamous Brushy Mountain State Prison, and the resources were extracted using prison labor. The logging era ended in the 1920s, and Frozen Head was declared a forest reserve. The Civilian Conservation Corps came in and established many of the trails that are in use today. A plaque at the main trailhead memorializes those who lost their lives developing the area. This is an ideal park for active people who like a small campground but want plenty of activities all within walking distance of the campground.

Frozen Head's campground is known as Big Cove Camping Area. A figure-eight loop contains 19 sites that border Big Cove Branch and Flat Fork Creek. Big Cove backs up to Bird Mountain and has a minor slope. The sites have been leveled and are set amid large boulders that came to rest untold eons ago after falling from Bird Mountain. The gray boulders strewn about give it a distinctive Cumberland Mountains feel. Second-growth

Emory Gap Falls is a beauty spot in Frozen Head State Park.

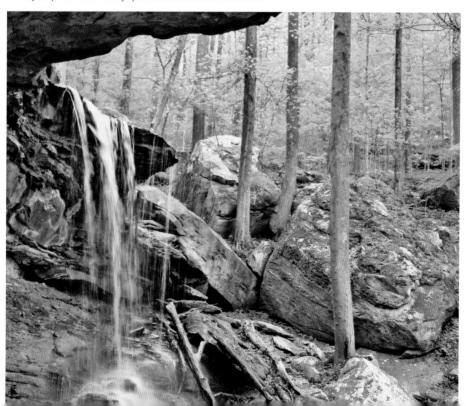

KEY INFORMATION

CONTACT: 423-346-3318, tnstateparks.com

OPEN: March 15–October

SITES: 20

EACH SITE HAS: Picnic table, fire grate with grill, lantern post

WHEELCHAIR ACCESS: One campsite

ASSIGNMENT: By reservation and daily walkup

REGISTRATION: At visitor center

AMENITIES: Water, flush toilets, hot showers

PARKING: At campsites and designated lots

FEES: $13.75/night

ELEVATION: 1,500'

RESTRICTIONS:

PETS: On leash only

QUIET HOURS: 10 p.m.–6 a.m.

FIRES: In fire grates only

ALCOHOL: Not allowed

VEHICLES: A narrow bridge crossing limits trailers to 16'

OTHER: 14-day stay limit

---

hardwoods provide ample shade, and the dogwood and hemlock understory allow some privacy for campers. The bathhouse is close to all, being in the middle of the campground. Single-sex hot showers and flush toilets are well maintained. Two spigots provide drinking water for the small campground.

Some sites are close together, but all provide enough room to spread out your gear. Two group sites are available and can be reserved. Ten sites allow tent and trailer camping; the other nine are for tents only. An overflow and off-season camping area sits along Flat Fork Creek up from the regular campground. It has only a camping spot and a fire ring. The park gates are closed from sunset to 8 a.m. Late-arriving campers must open and close the gate as they enter. It's best to get situated for the evening and stay within the park's confines. If you plan wisely, you won't even have to get back in your car until you leave for good; there's plenty to do. But if you forgot something, you can purchase supplies back in Wartburg, west on TN 62.

The trails of Frozen Head will take you to some fascinating places. The 3,324-foot Frozen Head observation tower is the apex of the trail system. You can see the surrounding highlands of the Cumberland Plateau and the Great Smoky Mountains in the distance. Other features include the Chimney Rock, a natural observation point that looks west as far as the eye can see. Or take the Panther Branch Trail 0.6 mile up to DeBord Falls. A mile farther is Emory Gap Falls. The Tower and Bird Mountain Trails leave directly from the campground. Two miles farther on the Bird Mountain Trail is one of Frozen Head's defining rock formations, Castle Rock. This rock formation is more than 100 feet high and 300 feet wide; with a little imagination, you can see the center edifice of the castle with turrets on both ends. These rock formations are the remnants of the erosion-resistant sandstone that covers the Cumberland Plateau. The softer rock and soil below this caprock eroded, leaving rock formations that seemingly jut straight out of the land. Bicyclers can stay on the Lookout Tower Trail and pedal all the way to the fire tower. Hikers can take this trail or one of many others for tower views.

If you don't feel like hiking or relaxing, there are many other activities. Play volleyball on one of the sand courts. Throw horseshoes in one of the three pits. Shoot some basketball at the outdoor court. Check out the free equipment you need at the park office. During the summer, the 240-seat amphitheater hosts many park activities, including interpretive talks, slide shows, movies, and music concerts.

I planned my trip to coincide with spring's wildflower display. Frozen Head has one of the richest wildflower areas in the Southeast. Even though I could observe purple, yellow, and white symbols of the season directly from my campground, I did tramp many stream-side trails and was glad that this piece of the Cumberlands was preserved for all to enjoy.

Frozen Head State Park Campground

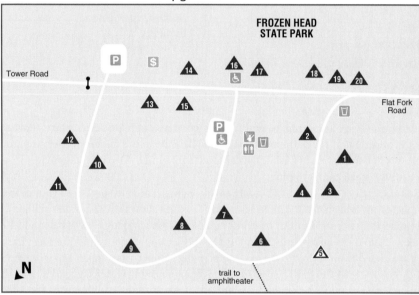

GETTING THERE

From Knoxville, take I-40 West for about 10 miles to Exit 376 (TN 162 North/Maryville/Oak Ridge). Merge onto TN 162 North, and drive 6.4 miles. Then merge onto TN 62 West, and drive 11.8 miles to Oliver Springs. Turn right to stay on TN 62 West, and drive 13.7 miles. At the sign for Frozen Head State Park, turn right onto Flat Fork Road, and drive about 4 miles to the park entrance. The visitor center will be on your right.

GPS COORDINATES N36° 07.836' W84° 29.880'

7

Hiwassee–Ocoee Scenic River State Park Campground

Beauty: ★★★★ Privacy: ★★★★ Spaciousness: ★★★★★ Quiet: ★★★ Security: ★★★★★ Cleanliness: ★★★★

It will take the Hiwassee River and the Gee Creek Wilderness to tear you away from this campground.

Known informally as Gee Creek Campground, the overnighting area of Hiwassee–Ocoee Scenic River State Park lies in a large, wooded flat at the base of Starr Mountain, adjacent to the cold, clear waters of the Hiwassee River. You can camp out in this high-quality destination and enjoy the Hiwassee River and the trails of the Cherokee National Forest, which abuts the state park. A tall pine forest once shaded the campground, but pine beetles decimated them. However, planted hardwoods are growing and providing shade.

The sites are widely spaced along two loops that meander amid the trees. The clean campsites are placed well apart from each other. Even without a lot of ground cover, the sheer number of trees and the distance between sites allow for adequate privacy. You never have to walk too far for water, as spigots are spread out along both loops. The campground is well maintained by state employees. A Tennessee State Park ranger lives opposite the campground.

The campground is open all year, yet it is heavily used only on summer weekends. The bathhouse is located near the center of the campground and is open from mid-March to the end of November. In winter, there are portable toilets, but showers are unavailable; drinking water is provided year-round.

Paddlers prepare to launch into the Hiwassee River.

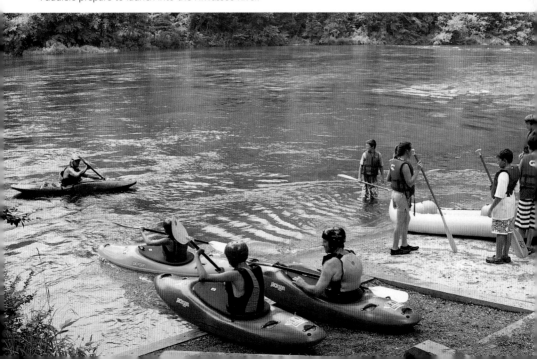

KEY INFORMATION

CONTACT: 423-263-0050, tnstateparks.com

OPEN: Year-round

SITES: 47

EACH SITE HAS: Picnic table, grill, fire pit, lantern post

WHEELCHAIR ACCESS: 2 sites

ASSIGNMENT: By reservation and daily walk-up

REGISTRATION: With park staff member on-site

AMENITIES: Drinking water, flush toilets, hot showers

PARKING: At campsites

FEES: $13.75/night

ELEVATION: 728'

RESTRICTIONS:

PETS: On leash only

QUIET HOURS: 10 p.m.–6 a.m.

FIRES: In fire rings only

ALCOHOL: Prohibited

VEHICLES: None

OTHER: 14-day stay limit

We visited during spring. Dogwoods bloomed above the needle-carpeted forest floor. Warm air and cool air played tug-of-war. Squirrels scampered about the campground. Birds flew purposefully from tree to tree. We could sense the rebirth of the mountains around us; it seemed leaves were greening and growing before our very eyes.

The Gee Creek Wilderness is a short distance away and certainly worth a visit. Drive back to US 411 and turn right, then turn right at the sign for Gee Creek after half a mile. Follow the paved road over the railroad tracks, then turn right. Drive 2 miles until the road turns to gravel. The Gee Creek Watchable Wildlife Trail is on your left. Just a short distance beyond that is the Gee Creek Trail itself. Trace the old angler's trail up the gorge. Multiple waterfalls provide plentiful photographic opportunities. The trail crosses the creek several times and dead-ends after 1.9 miles. On the return trip, look for the little things you missed on the way up. Skilled rock climbers can climb some of the creekside bluffs.

The Gee Creek Watchable Wildlife Trail is a 0.7-mile trail designed to increase the hiker's knowledge of nature's signs. The U.S. Forest Service has placed nest boxes, interpretive information, and wildlife plantings; they have also made a track pit to see which animals have passed by. This is an excellent trail to get children interested in nature. Also starting at the Gee Creek trailhead is the Starr Mountain Trail. It leads 4.8 miles up to the ridgeline of Starr Mountain and offers expansive views of the surrounding area. The John Muir Trail cruises upstream along the Hiwassee for more than 20 miles, starting just east of the TN 315 bridge over the river near Reliance. It offers not only quality hiking but also fishing accesses.

After all this hiking, maybe you need to cool down. Why not enjoy the Hiwassee River? Draining more than 750,000 acres of forested mountain land, it has clear, pure water. Informal trails lead to and along the river from the campground. Make sure young children are supervised. When the turbines upstream are generating, the water will be swift. Most water lovers enjoy the river by raft, canoe, funyak (inflatable kayak), or tube. It's a 5.5-mile float through the splendid Cherokee National Forest. The Hiwassee, a State Scenic River, is primarily Class I and II on the international scale of difficulty and is very cold. Outfitters will supply anything you need, including a shuttle up the river if you have your own equipment. I recommend Hiwassee Outfitters, a reputable family operation (hiwasseeoutfitters.com).

The nearby Ocoee River has more challenging whitewater. Bevies of outfitters operate the river and will guide you through the exciting whitewater rapids.

The Hiwassee is also a mecca for those hoping to catch trout. Anglers head to the river on foggy mornings to toss their flies before unsuspecting trout. If you want to try your luck and are ill prepared, there are stores and outfitters nearby who will get you on or in the water. The old train depot town of Etowah is 6 miles north on US 411 if you need supplies.

Hiwassee–Ocoee Scenic River State Park Campground

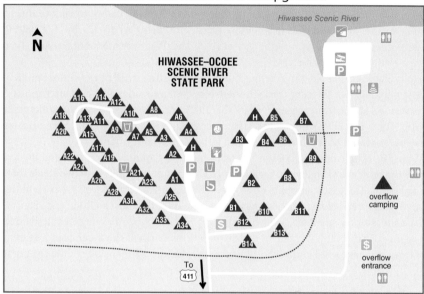

GETTING THERE

From I-75, take Exit 36 (TN 163/Calhoun). Turn onto TN 163 East, following signs for Hiwassee–Ocoee State Park. Drive 2.3 miles, then turn right onto US 11 South, and drive 0.6 mile. Turn left onto TN 163, and drive 13 miles. Turn right onto US 411 South, and drive 0.9 mile. Turn left onto Spring Creek Road, and drive 1.1 miles; then turn right into the campground.

GPS COORDINATES N35° 14.047' W84° 32.962'

8

⛺ Holly Flats Campground

Beauty: ★★★★ Privacy: ★★★★ Spaciousness: ★★★★★ Quiet: ★★★★★ Security: ★★ Cleanliness: ★★★

Shoes are a must in this old-time campground next door to the Bald River Wilderness.

If you place a high priority on barefoot tent camping, skip Holly Flats. True to its name, the cozy Holly Flats Campground is dotted by holly trees shedding their prickly leaves on the woodland floor. But if you don't mind wearing shoes while you camp, you'll love this place. It offers a variety of campsites in a remote place with plenty to do nearby. The Bald River Gorge Wilderness is just across the gravel road, and Waucheesi Mountain and Warriors Passage National Recreation Trail are close as well.

Holly Flats has that old-time campground ambience: the smell of wood smoke and hamburgers cooking; sun filtering through the trees; cool mornings and lazy afternoons. This timeworn feel stems from the simple fact that the campground is old. Think antique. Think historic. Think classic. It's not all bad. The campground is like an old pair of favorite shoes: it may be worn and have a few scuff marks, but it sure is comfortable.

Cross the bridge over Bald River to reach the campground. Two sites stand in a grassy area by the bridge for sun lovers. Farther up, the campground splits into two roads that end in small loops. The first road splits off to the right, away from Bald River. It has eight thickly wooded sites spread along a small ridge. These sites offer the most solitude and silence. The farthest site is atop a small hill, away from the road. The second road runs next to Bald River. All six sites are directly riverside in a narrow flat. More open, these campsites lie beneath large trees and have a holly-and-rhododendron understory. The melody of the river making

The author admires waterfalls in the Bald River Gorge Wilderness.

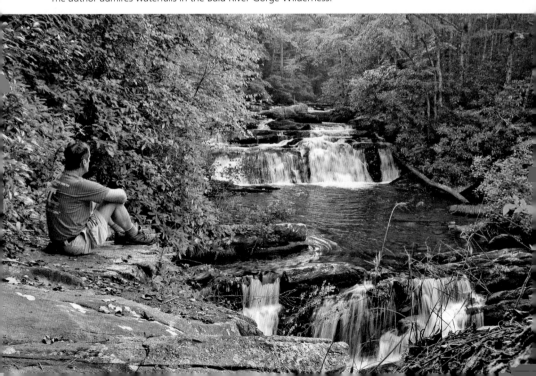

KEY INFORMATION

CONTACT: 423-253-8400, www.fs.usda.gov
/cherokee

OPEN: Mid-March–mid-September

SITES: 16

EACH SITE HAS: Tent pad, picnic table,
fire ring

WHEELCHAIR ACCESS: Some sites

ASSIGNMENT: First-come, first-served;
no reservations

REGISTRATION: Self-register on-site

AMENITIES: Vault toilet

PARKING: At campsites only

FEES: $6/night

ELEVATION: 2,150'

RESTRICTIONS:

PETS: On leash only

QUIET HOURS: 10 p.m.–6 a.m.

FIRES: In fire rings only

ALCOHOL: At campsites only

VEHICLES: Parking at sites only

OTHER: Pack it in, pack it out

---

its descent pervades the flat. A comfort station with vault toilets for each sex is on the side of the road opposite Bald River. Holly Flats is a designated pack-it-in, pack-it-out campground. It has no trash receptacles. Pack out all your trash and any trash that thoughtless campers left behind. Bring your own water, too.

Several hiking trails start near Holly Flats. The Bald River Trail (88) starts 0.4 mile west down the Bald River on Forest Service Road 126 and strikes through the heart of the 3,700-acre Bald River Gorge Wilderness. The trail leads 4.8 miles through the steep-sided gorge, passing lesser falls en route to grand Bald River Falls, making for an excellent day hike. For those interested in angling, Bald River is a noted trout stream.

The Kirkland Creek Trail (85) starts 0.4 mile east of the campground on FS 126. A variety of forest types are represented along its route. The trail follows a stream and runs up a valley for 3 miles, then follows an old logging road to Sandy Gap and the North Carolina state line at 4.6 miles.

Less than 1 mile east of Holly Flats on FS 126 is the Brookshire Creek Trail (180). It starts in an old field, crosses Bald River, and climbs 6 miles to the state line. Brookshire Creek offers quality trout fishing as well. Upper Bald River Falls crashes 2.4 miles from the trailhead. Also up the trail are some very remote old homesites where, in times past, subsistence mountain farmers cultivated the hills and battled the elements to carve out a living. To get a sweat-free overlay of the land, drive to the top of 3,692-foot Waucheesi Mountain. Rangers formerly watched for fires from an old tower there. Although the tower has since been torn down, one can still get a view from ground level. From Holly Flats drive west on FS 126 to FS 126C. Turn left and climb the mountain; FS 126C ends at the top. You can peer down into the Bald River Gorge and the Tellico River basin. The Warriors Passage National Recreation Trail (164) starts partway up FS 126C on your right. The trail traces an old route used by the Cherokee on their travels between settlements and, later, by white traders and soldiers who eventually drove the Cherokee out. The historic trail leads to FS 76, 5 miles away. Holly Flats is a relaxing campground bordering one of Tennessee's finest wilderness areas. This part of the Cherokee National Forest is worth a look—and a night or two tent camping at Holly Flats.

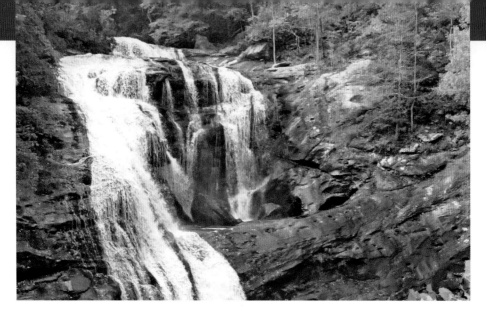

Bald River Falls

Holly Flats Campground

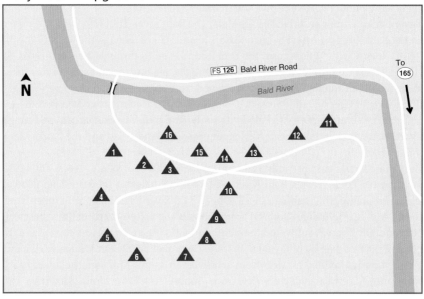

GETTING THERE

From I-75, take Exit 60 (TN 68/Sweetwater/Spring City), and turn onto TN 68 South. Drive 24.2 miles to Tellico Plains. Turn left onto TN 165 East/Cherohala Skyway/Unicoi Turnpike, and drive 5.2 miles. Turn right onto River Road, and drive 13.8 miles. Turn right onto FS 126, and drive 5.6 miles. Holly Flats Campground will be across a bridge on your left.

GPS COORDINATES N35° 17.092' W84° 10.742'

9

Indian Boundary Campground

Beauty: ★★★★★ Privacy: ★★★ Spaciousness: ★★★ Quiet: ★★★★ Security: ★★★★ Cleanliness: ★★★★

Indian Boundary is the pride of the Cherokee National Forest.

Indian Boundary is the pride of the southern Cherokee National Forest. And with good reason—the wooded camping area lies in a flat beside a clear lake and is overlooked by mountain splendor. Individual campsites are tastefully integrated into the natural beauty of the land adjacent to Flats Mountain. Nearby recreational opportunities center around, but are not limited to, Indian Boundary Lake. The campground is an excellent choice for campers who want a scenic setting, a campground with amenities, and plenty of land- and water-based activities.

The main campground is divided into four loops. Loop A is closest to Indian Boundary Lake. A pine-and-oak forest cloaks the rolling hills here, making for a good combination of sun and shade. As with all the loops, a campground host is there to help campers enjoy their stay. Two comfort stations here have warm showers.

A lone boat waits for someone to paddle it into autumn's glory.

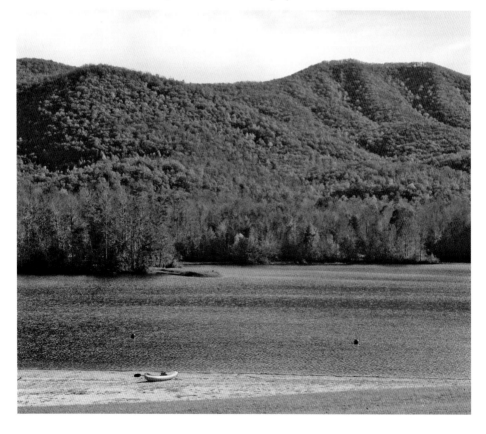

KEY INFORMATION

CONTACT: 423-253-2520, www.fs.usda.gov
/cherokee; reservations: 877-444-6777,
recreation.gov

OPEN: Main campground, late-April–early
November; overflow area, year-round

SITES: 87

EACH SITE HAS: Picnic table, fire grate,
lantern post, electricity, water

WHEELCHAIR ACCESS: Some sites

ASSIGNMENT: First-come, first-served and
by reservation

REGISTRATION: On-site

AMENITIES: Showers, flush toilets, camp store

PARKING: At campsites only

FEES: $20/night

ELEVATION: 1,800'

RESTRICTIONS:

PETS: On leash only

QUIET HOURS: 10 p.m.–6 a.m.

FIRES: In fire grates only

ALCOHOL: At campsites only

VEHICLES: 25' length limit

OTHER: 14-day stay limit

Loop B is shaded by tall white pines and oaks. Loop C and Loop D interconnect beneath rolling pine woods bisected by a small creek bed, but they are farthest from the lake, which is the focus of recreation here. Anglers enjoy bank fishing or launching a boat into the clear waters here. The atmosphere stays quiet because no gas motors are allowed. The view of the surrounding mountains from the lake may distract anglers from vying for largemouth bass, trout, and bream or the tackle-busting catfish that purportedly wait down deep. A swimming beach extends along one section of the impoundment. The Lakeshore Trail makes a 3.2-mile loop around Indian Boundary Lake, which delivers aquatic vistas as well as montane moments.

More-ambitious hikers have the Citico Creek Wilderness in which to tramp. Just a piece down Forest Service Road 35-1 is the South Fork Citico Creek trailhead. Here, hikers can make loops involving the Brush Mountain, Pine Ridge, and North and South Fork Citico Creek Trails. Stream anglers can enjoy the wild setting while casting a line for native trout in Citico Creek and its tributaries. Order a map of the Citico Creek Wilderness before you come.

Campers reach Indian Boundary via the Cherohala Skyway. This scenic road rivals the Blue Ridge Parkway or Newfound Gap Road in the Smokies for scenery. Uphill from Indian Boundary, scenic overlooks dot the way to Beech Gap and beyond the North Carolina state line. Also at Beech Gap is the Fodderstack Trail. This path traces an old road for a distance then climbs up to Bob Bald, a mile-high open meadow. An easier hike is the one to Hooper Bald; the trail lies a little farther along the Cherohala Skyway. Take a short nature trail to reach this meadow at 5,300 feet. More views await at nearby Huckleberry Knob. For more information about the scenic road, visit cherohala.org.

Indian Boundary is a popular destination. Expect a full campground during the peak summer season. The reservation system can guarantee you a campsite. There are less crowded times to visit, though. Consider coming here in May. Fall is also a good choice; leaf viewers are likely to see vibrant colors, since the Cherohala Skyway traverses elevations from less than 1,000 feet to more than 5,000 feet. No matter what time of year, you should head for the borders of Indian Boundary.

Indian Boundary Campground

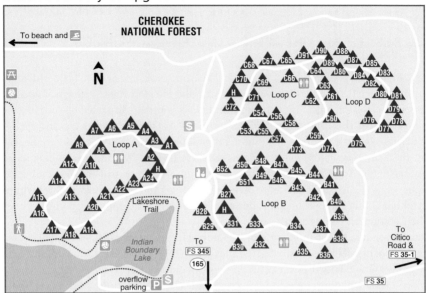

GETTING THERE

From I-75, take Exit 60 (TN 68/Sweetwater/Spring City), and turn onto TN 68 South. Drive 24.2 miles to Tellico Plains. Turn left onto TN 165 East/Cherohala Skyway/Unicoi Turnpike, and drive 14.3 miles. Turn left onto Forest Service Road 345/Indian Boundary Road, and drive 1.3 miles to the campground.

GPS COORDINATES N35° 23.825' W84° 06.396'

Indian Boundary Lake from Cherohala Skyway *Photo: Martha Marks/Shutterstock*

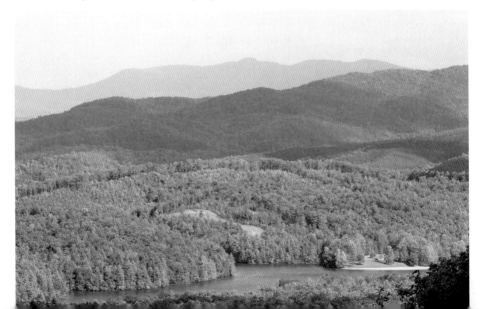

10

⛺ Little Oak Campground

Beauty: ★★★★ Privacy: ★★★★ Spaciousness: ★★★★★ Quiet: ★★★ Security: ★★★★★ Cleanliness: ★★★★

Picking the best of these sites will be your biggest problem at Little Oak.

Lakeside camping is a breeze at Little Oak. The camp is sizable and well laid out, situated atop what was left of Little Oak Mountain after the Holston River Valley was flooded to create South Holston Lake. Though large, Little Oak is widely dispersed on four loops that jut into the lake. This arrangement allows for many spacious lakeside sites, and each loop feels like its own little campground. Short paths slope from each lakeside site to the water's edge. There are many attractive sites from which to choose. We drove each loop so many times, seeing one ideal site and then seeing an even better one, that we were sure another camper was going to turn our license plate in to a ranger (note your favorite sites with your smartphone). This campground was designed for a pleasant camping experience, not just as a way station for the urban masses.

Just beyond the pay station is Hemlock Loop, which contains 14 sites nestled beneath a thick stand of hemlock trees. Most of the sites are on the outside of the loop, well away from one another, with plenty of cover between sites. An old-fashioned vault toilet and a modern comfort station with flush toilets and showers are at the head of the loop. Camp at Hemlock Loop if you like very shady sites.

Misty fall view of South Holston Lake

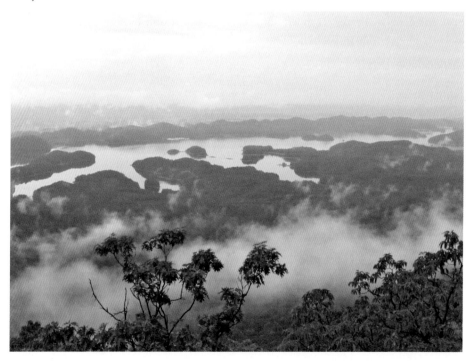

KEY INFORMATION

CONTACT: 423-735-1500, www.fs.usda.gov
/cherokee; reservations: 877-444-6777,
recreation.gov

OPEN: April–mid-November

SITES: 72

EACH SITE HAS: Tent pad, picnic table, fire
ring, lantern post

WHEELCHAIR ACCESS: Some sites

ASSIGNMENT: First-come, first-served and
by reservation

REGISTRATION: Self-register on-site

AMENITIES: Water faucets, flush toilets,
warm showers

PARKING: At campsites only

FEES: $12/night, $10 when running water
is unavailable

ELEVATION: 1,750'

RESTRICTIONS:

PETS: On leash only

QUIET HOURS: 10 p.m.–6 a.m.

FIRES: In fire rings only

ALCOHOL: Prohibited

VEHICLES: None

OTHER: 14-day stay limit

Lone Pine Loop is for those who prefer sunny sites. Two small fields adjacent to the loop allow more light into the camping areas. Three comfort stations are located by the 16 sites. Only the northern end of the loop has lakeside sites.

Big Oak Loop has 16 sites and is located on a spit of hardwoods and evergreens that juts north into the lake. Nearly all the sites are lakeside. A modern comfort station is located halfway along the loop, and water faucets are nearby. The view from Big Oak Loop into South Holston Lake is my personal favorite.

Poplar Loop is the largest loop, with 23 sites, but the sites are split into two loops of their own, facing west and south into the lake. There is a modern comfort station at each loop. Most of these sites are lakeside.

We finally settled on Big Oak Loop. After setting up camp, we watched the sun turn into a red ball of fire over South Holston Lake. Gentle waves lapped at our feet as we sat on the shoreline. We took a vigorous hike in the cool of the next morning on the Little Oak Trail that loops the outer peninsula of the campground. This campground is virtually surrounded by the lake, which lends an aquatic ambience. For a different perspective, take the Little Oak Mountain Trail. It leaves the campground near the pay station and circles back after dipping into the woods. For yet another perspective on Little Oak, get out on the lake itself. A boat ramp is conveniently situated between the Hemlock and Poplar Loops. Swim, fish, or take a pleasure ride up the lake into Virginia. Bring your canoe or kayak for a slower, more relaxing experience.

In East Tennessee, the high country is never far away. Little Oak is near the Flint Mill Scenic Area, which features a broad representation of Southern Appalachian flora and fauna—elevations exceeding 4,000 feet. Turn right out of the campground onto Forest Service Road 87 and drive a short 1.4 miles. The Josiah Trail (Forest Trail 50) starts on your left and ascends 2.2 miles to a saddle on Holston Mountain and Forest Trail 44. Flint Mill Trail (Forest Trail 49) climbs one steep mile to Flint Rock and some fantastic views of South Holston Lake—you can even see Little Oak Campground! The trail is 2.2 miles on the left beyond the Josiah Trail. Fishing equipment and other supplies are available back in Bristol.

Little Oak Campground

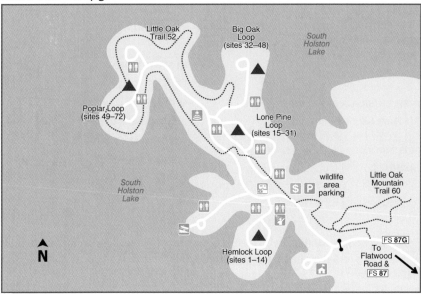

GETTING THERE

From I-81 in Virginia, take Exit 3 (I-381 South/Bristol). Drive 2.4 miles (I-381 South will become Commonwealth Avenue and then Volunteer Parkway); then turn left onto Anderson Street, and drive 1.5 miles (Anderson Street will become Pennsylvania Avenue). Turn left onto East Cedar Street, and drive just 0.1 mile; then turn right onto Virginia Avenue/US 421 South, and drive 13.4 miles. Turn right onto Camp Tom Howard Road/FS 87, and continue on FS 87 for 6.6 miles. Turn right onto Little Oak Road/FS 87G, and drive about 1.5 miles to dead-end into Little Oak Recreation Area.

GPS COORDINATES N36° 31.304' W82° 03.883'

11

Nolichucky Gorge Campground and Cabins

Beauty: ★★★★ Privacy: ★★★ Spaciousness: ★★★★ Quiet: ★★★★ Security: ★★★★ Cleanliness: ★★★★★

Raft, hike, fish, and camp in the deep gorge of the Nolichucky River.

The Nolichucky River cuts a deep gorge through the Appalachian Mountains as it flows from North Carolina into Tennessee. Frothing whitewater tumbles over rocks and boulders beneath towering green ridges. Just a short distance into the Volunteer State, Jones Branch flows into the Nolichucky, creating a riverside flat where Rick Murray, rafter and whitewater man extraordinaire, located his Nolichucky Gorge Campground. This flat, overlooking the river, is surrounded by national forest land, with the exception of a rafting company located next door. Having such a neighbor enhances the camping experience here, as rafting the Nolichucky is the primary recreational activity in the gorge. Furthermore, the Appalachian Trail (AT) passes a mere 50 yards no your campsite, offering hiking opportunities. One more thing: the fishing here can be very good.

Let's start with the campground. Cross Jones Branch on a small bridge and enter the camping area. Along the creek are six shaded RV campsites. To the right is the Nolichucky River.; here, six tent sites that offer ideal access and even better views of the mountains beyond are stretched along the water. Some sites are shaded; others are more in the open. A grassy lawn provides the understory. To your left is a gravel loop road. Here are the campground office, six more RV sites, and two cabins that are mostly in the open. Backing up to the hillside are five more shaded tent sites. Also back here are two more cabins deep in the

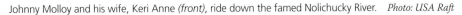

Johnny Molloy and his wife, Keri Anne *(front)*, ride down the famed Nolichucky River. *Photo: USA Raft*

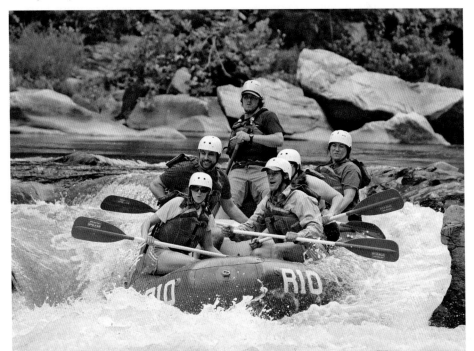

KEY INFORMATION

CONTACT: 423-743-8876, nolichucky.com

OPEN: Year-round

SITES: 31 tent sites (approximate) and 12 RV sites, plus 4 cabins

EACH SITE HAS: Picnic table, fire ring

WHEELCHAIR ACCESS: None

ASSIGNMENT: First-come, first-served

REGISTRATION: At campground office

AMENITIES: Hot showers, flush toilets, water spigots

PARKING: At campsites only

FEES: $12 tent sites, $40 RV sites, $69–$219 cabins, $5 kids ages 6–13, free for kids age 12 and younger, $4 day-use fee. Prices are per person, per night, except for RV sites, which are for 2 people/night (+ $10/night for each additional person). Seventh night is free.

ELEVATION: 1,750'

RESTRICTIONS:

PETS: On leash 6' or shorter

FIRES: In fire rings only

QUIET HOURS: 11 p.m.–7 a.m.

ALCOHOL: At campsites only

VEHICLES: None

---

shade of pine and tulip trees. Deep in more pines is an open tenting area; the sites aren't defined, but shade lovers will snap them up.

An open understory diminishes campsite privacy. Most sites rate above average on spaciousness. Nolichucky Gorge encourages reservations, and I do too—when the river is running, the campground can fill because the Nolichucky Gorge is all about whitewater.

The primary rafting run starts in North Carolina, 9 miles upstream. This run offers Class III and IV whitewater and *gorge*-ous scenery. The Noli, as it is known among whitewater aficionados, streams from the slopes of Mount Mitchell, the highest point in the East, and slices through the Unaka Mountains. The Unakas are mostly forested, with serrated outcrops of stone jutting above the wood. Being on national forest land gives the river run a wild and natural aura. Many folks bring their own kayaks and whitewater canoes. Increasing in popularity these days are "funyaks," or inflatable kayaks. If you don't have your own boat, walk across Jones Branch to USA Raft (800-872-7238, usaraft.com). This rafting company uses self-bailing rafts that drain the water as it splashes overboard. You can also tube downstream from the campground in milder water that is primarily Class II in difficulty.

You can enjoy the water without a boat as well. Take a trail from the campground heading upstream along the river to the campground swimming beach. This way you can intentionally take a dip instead of taking one falling overboard. You can also fish the Nolichucky; trout swim the refreshing waters, as do smallmouth bass, catfish, and muskellunge.

Land-based recreation focuses on the AT. Southbound hikers can wind their way along the steep cliffs of the Nolichucky Gorge 1.3 miles to reach the bridge crossing the river over which you drove to get to the campground. It's a steep climb if you keep going, but you'll be rewarded with fine views of the Nolichucky Gorge. Northbound hikers will ascend from the river to eventually reach the Curley Maple Gap Shelter after 3 miles and Indian Grave Gap 4 miles beyond that. (Unless you have a backpack and sleeping bag, you'll have a hard time making it all the way to Maine.) Other hikers wend their way up the banks of the Nolichucky, exploring the streamside finery. So head on back to the Nolichucky Gorge, a fine place to be, whether you're hiking, fishing, or rafting.

Nolichucky Gorge Campground and Cabins

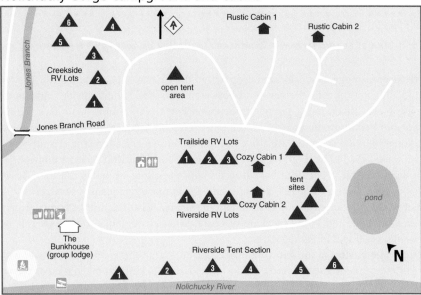

GETTING THERE

From I-26, take Exit 40 (Jackson Love Highway/Erwin). Turn onto TN 36 South—a right turn from I-26 West or a left turn from I-26 East—and then take the very next right onto Temple Hill Road. Drive 0.8 mile; then turn left onto River Road/Unaka Springs Road, and drive 0.5 mile. Turn left onto Chestoa Pike, and drive just 0.1 mile over the Nolichucky River; then turn right onto Jones Branch Road, and drive 1.2 miles to dead-end at the campground, just beyond the rafting center.

GPS COORDINATES N36° 05.915' W82° 25.899'

12

North River Campground

Beauty: ★★★★★ Privacy: ★★★★ Spaciousness: ★★★★★ Quiet: ★★★★ Security: ★★★ Cleanliness: ★★★

Let this slice of scenic stream in Southern Appalachia be your quiet woodland escape.

North River Campground is located deep within the Cherokee National Forest. The campground, situated on a level river bend between a wooded mountainside and the clear-running North River, has a serene atmosphere. For a tent camper who likes minimum fanfare and maximum nature, this is the place. Human accoutrements are sparse in this U.S. Forest Service camping area, but natural amenities are abundant. Trout swim the creek's waters shaded by tulip trees, sycamore, and rhododendron. Mature dogwoods and white pine provide a beautiful backdrop for those relaxing evenings fireside. There are grassy areas between the trees, accentuating the ample spaciousness between the level tent sites. Dead, fallen firewood is abundant in the area, as are nature's citizens: deer, wild turkey, wild boar, and bear (Speaking of bears, safely store your food unless it is being eaten—it's a national forest regulation).

With only 11 sites in the entire campground, quiet rules here. The North River will lull you to sleep at night and the birds will be your alarm clock in the morning. For the water lover, 8 of the 11 sites are riverside. Two of the sites could qualify as group sites, with double picnic tables, additional tent pads, and ample parking for families. In contrast, the lower end of the campground is shadier and more isolated, while the upper end is sunnier and more open. Bathroom facilities are spartan, with one pit toilet for each sex. If the amenities sound too coarse, remember that this is a place to come to relish the out-of-doors and a bygone way of life vanishing in our digital age.

A stretch of the upper North River

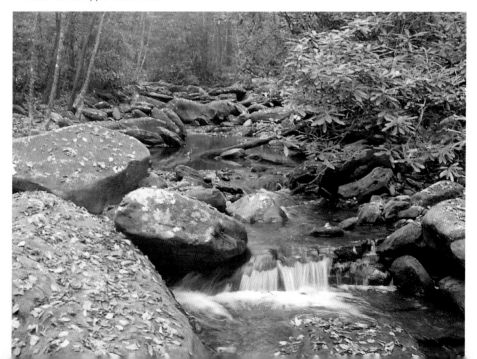

KEY INFORMATION

CONTACT: 423-253-8400, www.fs.usda.gov
  /cherokee

OPEN: Mid-March–October

SITES: 11

EACH SITE HAS: Graveled tent pad, picnic
  table, fire ring, lantern holder

WHEELCHAIR ACCESS: Some sites

ASSIGNMENT: First-come, first-served;
  no reservations

REGISTRATION: Self-register on-site

AMENITIES: Pit toilet

PARKING: At campsites only

FEES: $8/night

ELEVATION: 1,840'

RESTRICTIONS:

PETS: On leash or under physical control

QUIET HOURS: 10 p.m.–6 a.m.

FIRES: In fire rings only

ALCOHOL: At campsites only

VEHICLES: At campsites only

OTHER: 14-day stay limit

Beard cane, a species of grass, grows alongside the North River in the campground. The leaves on the main stem of the cane form the plant's "beard." Mountaineers once used the plant for fishing poles. Modern-day anglers prefer to fly-fish and are inspired by a trip to the nearby Pheasant Fields Fish Hatchery, 4.5 miles away. Turn right out of the campground and turn right again 0.1 mile down Forest Service Road 216. Go 1 mile and turn left up FS 210, then travel 3.5 miles. Rainbow trout are raised at the hatchery for stocking, and in one of the many tanks, there are some lunkers that will cause your eyes to pop in disbelief.

If you get the urge to explore, stretch your legs on the Sycamore Creek Trail (Forest Trail 61), which starts at the fish hatchery. Sycamore Creek is the feeder stream for the hatchery. The trail leads up to Whigg Meadow, an open field nearly a mile high, sporting views into Citico Creek and Slickrock Wilderness. Nearby, down FS 217 from the campground, are the McNabb and Hemlock Creek Trails (92 and 101, respectively). These trails are located in the Brushy Ridge Primitive Area just across from the campground. Each footpath follows a scenic tributary of the North River up to the high country. Before darkness falls, grab your smartphone and drive back to Bald River Falls for some scenic shots of this panoramic waterfall.

While exploring the area, my friends and I came to a rough road a few miles beyond the hatchery, just over the North Carolina line. We followed it for a distance because I wanted to show them where I had become stuck fording the Tellico River. As we came upon the crossing, we found a frustrated couple standing by their four-wheel-drive vehicle: it was stuck in the very place that mine had been stuck a decade earlier! We pulled them out with a chain and turned around, laughing at the irony of the situation.

During the summer, you can purchase supplies in the small community of Green Cove. It is an inholding in the national forest, consisting of summer cottages, a little motel, a small country store, and a gas station. Green Cove is located 2 miles from the campground up FS 210 before the fish hatchery.

If you want to camp in a national forest surrounded by natural beauty, come to the North River Campground. Literally encircled by mountainous woodland, it is spacious enough that you never feel packed in. Fellow campers are likely to be friendly locals from Monroe County who will help you in any way they can.

North River Campground

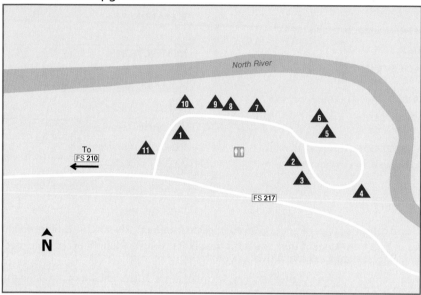

GETTING THERE

From I-75, take Exit 60 (TN 68/Sweetwater/Spring City), and turn onto TN 68 South. Drive 24.2 miles to Tellico Plains. Turn left onto TN 165 East/Cherohala Skyway/Unicoi Turnpike, and drive 5.2 miles. Turn right onto River Road, and drive 11.8 miles (you'll pass Baldy River Falls at 6.3 miles). Turn left onto FS 217, and drive 0.8 mile to the campground, on your right.

GPS COORDINATES N35° 19.103' W84° 07.431'

13

Obed Wild and Scenic River: Rock Creek Campground

Beauty: ★★★★★ Privacy: ★★★ Spaciousness: ★★★ Quiet: ★★★★ Security: ★★★ Cleanliness: ★★★

Enjoy the wonders of the wild and scenic Obed River from this campground.

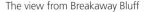

The Obed Wild and Scenic River, administered by the National Park Service, has come of age. What was once a protected recreation area in name only has now evolved into a multiple-outdoor-activity destination supported by the community. It all began with die-hard kayakers and canoers plying the whitewater of the Obed–Emory River watershed. Next, a few paddle access points were established. Then a 14-mile segment of the Cumberland Trail, which runs through the heart of the Obed River gorge, was completed. The addition of Rock Creek Campground at the Nemo Bridge boat access has made this scenic swath of the Cumberland Plateau a prime destination for tent campers.

When I started coming here over two decades ago, the Nemo Bridge area was a local party spot. Boy, have things changed. The old boat access is now a nice picnic area and trailhead. And the campground itself has been rehabbed, with new picnic tables, improved tent pads, and restrooms. The old Nemo Bridge is used for foot traffic only. Continue across the new bridge, turn right, and descend into the campground after crossing clear Rock Creek. Dead ahead is the self-service fee station. To the left is a single campsite that offers the most privacy. Enter tall woodland of sycamore and tulip trees, and pass the Cumberland Trail, which conveniently leaves directly from the camping area. One site lies near the trail. Pass two vault toilets, and then come to two nice campsites that are just a stone's throw from the Obed River. A nature trail heads upriver beyond these two campsites.

The view from Breakaway Bluff

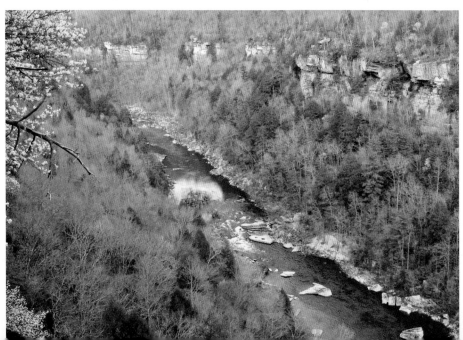

KEY INFORMATION

CONTACT: 423-346-6294, nps.gov/obed;
reservations: 877-444-6777, recreation.gov

OPEN: Year-round

SITES: 12

EACH SITE HAS: Picnic table, fire ring,
lantern post, tent pad, bearproof food-
storage lockers

ASSIGNMENT: By reservation only

WHEELCHAIR ACCESS: Yes, 1 campsite

REGISTRATION: Online

AMENITIES: Vault toilets, bring your
own water

PARKING: At campsites and overflow lots

FEES: $10/night

ELEVATION: 900'

RESTRICTIONS:

PETS: On leash 6' or shorter

QUIET HOURS: 10 p.m.–6 a.m.

FIRES: In fire rings only

ALCOHOL: At campsites only

VEHICLES: Maximum 2 vehicles/site

OTHER: 14-day stay limit

The high-quality design of Rock Creek Campground is immediately evident, with the landscaping timbers delineating the sites, which have raised tent pads that offer quick drainage and easy staking. The fire rings and lantern posts are placed to last a long time. Curve along the river and come to campsite 5. It is also close to the river and near Rock Creek as well. Pass two more good sites; then come to a set of three walk-in tent campsites. Two wooden bridges span a wet-weather drainage to access the shady sites that feature some hemlocks and rhododendron. The final site is wheelchair accessible.

All sites must be reserved through Recreation.gov (see Key Information). Getting a site is no problem during the week and in the fall and winter. Summer weekdays are good too. Plan to scramble for a site on spring weekends when the water is right for paddling.

So what about all the great recreation here? The Obed actually consists of four drainages that offer paddling of all difficulties. These watercourses—Daddys Creek, Clear Creek, Emory River, and the Obed River—have cut gorges into the Cumberland Plateau, where bluffs overlook rock-choked rivers running through thick forests. Upper Daddys Creek is for experts only, but the last 2 miles, from the Devils Breakfast Table onward are Class II water, as is the Emory River from Nemo Bridge to Oakdale, which takes one across the park's boundary. Just watch for that first rapid, Nemo: it has flipped me a few times. Some sections of Clear Creek are doable by average boaters, but other runs are tough. If you are going to paddle, on your initial trips go with someone who knows the water, and call the visitor center for water levels.

The rivers are good for fishing too. Muskie, bass, bream, and catfish await in the river's deeper holes; most of these are accessible by self-propelled boat or foot only. This National Park Service destination also has a good walk for you: Take the Cumberland Trail from the campground up the Emory River, climbing away from the water before it reaches its confluence with the Obed. At 2.6 miles, you will near Alley Ford. Another 2 miles will take you to Breakaway Bluff Overlook. The trail travels on to Rock Garden Overlook and views of rapids before picking up an old railroad bed. The 14-mile trail ends at the Devils Breakfast Table on Daddys Creek. If this one-way trek is too far, consider driving to the Devils Breakfast Table and starting down Daddys Creek, where two overlooks await in the first mile. The Rain House, a rock shelter, is a mile farther on. Pick up a trail map and park map at the visitor center in Wartburg or download one ahead of time. A shorter option is taking the Cumberland Trail up the Emory to a nature trail that leaves right and descends to end at the campground, near the water's edge. No matter which option you choose, grab your tent and head for the Obed.

Obed Wild and Scenic River: Rock Creek Campground

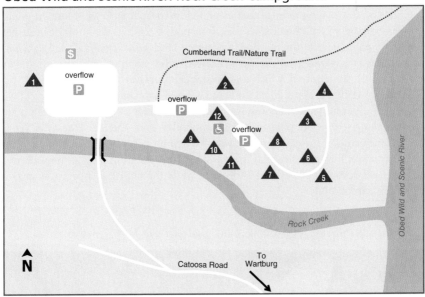

GETTING THERE

From I-40, take Exit 347 (US 27/Harriman/Rockwood). Turn right onto US 27 North, and drive 6.5 miles. Keep left to stay on US 27 North, and drive 12.3 miles to Wartburg. Turn left onto Main Street, and drive 1.1 miles, then turn left onto South Church Street (or turn right one block before, at Maiden Street, to detour to the Obed Visitor Center, one block north). At the next intersection, turn right onto Spring Street, and drive 0.2 mile; then turn left onto Catoosa Road, and drive 5.6 miles. The campground will be on your right, just past the bridge over the Emory River.

GPS COORDINATES N36° 04.146' W84° 39.777'

14

Old Forge Campground

Beauty: ★★★★ Privacy: ★★★ Spaciousness: ★★★★ Quiet: ★★★★★ Security: ★★★ Cleanliness: ★★★

Old Forge has been melded into a model tenter's campground.

Old Forge was the site of an iron forge in the early 1900s. Iron was melted and made into tools for use on the logging railroad that extended up to Cold Springs Mountain. Men cut the timber by hand with crosscut saws then transported the logs via horse or mule before loading them onto trains at the railroad. Talk about hard work! That makes it all the more ironic that this is a recreational site now. It doesn't take much effort nowadays to have a good time at this campground, which was revamped exclusively for tent campers.

The natural setting is appealing. Old Forge is set in a flat along Jennings Creek, which tumbles into numerous falls and pools, some large enough for a swim. Overhead is a mix of hardwoods along with white pine and a little rhododendron. The U.S. Forest Service built a wooden fence around the campground with handsome archway entrances. Pass through the archway and follow a gravel path from which little spur trails lead to the walk-in tent campsites. Tent campers are grouped together, while the big-rig campers stay at nearby Horse Creek Campground.

The trails emanating from Old Forge make for prime wildflower hikes.

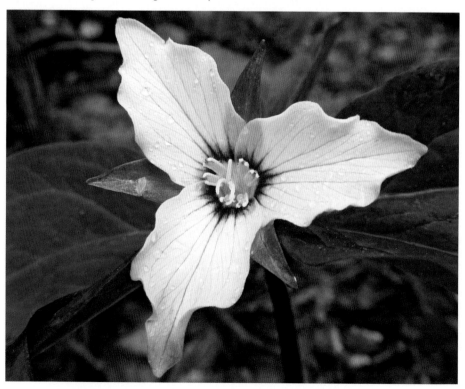

KEY INFORMATION

CONTACT: 423-638-4109, www.fs.usda.gov
/cherokee

OPEN: April–mid-December

SITES: 10

EACH SITE HAS: Picnic table, fire ring,
lantern post, tent pad

WHEELCHAIR ACCESS: One campsite
Assignment: First-come, first-served;
no reservations

REGISTRATION: Self-register on-site

AMENITIES: Vault toilet

PARKING: At tent-camper parking only

FEES: $7/night

ELEVATION: 1,920'

RESTRICTIONS:

PETS: On leash only

QUIET HOURS: 10 p.m.–6 a.m.

FIRES: In fire rings only

ALCOHOL: Not allowed

VEHICLES: None

OTHER: 14-day stay limit

Swing up the flat and pass a few sites that are farther away from the creek but closest to the parking area. Three sites at the head of the flat offer lush solitude. These are ideal campsites for hikers, as they are closest to an archway leading out of the camp onto the Bald Mountain Ridge Scenic Area's trail system. The campground path then swings alongside Jennings Creek, passing the five waterside sites. A couple of spur paths lead down to waterfall overlooks and big pools on the moderate-size stream. One campsite is all by its lonesome self, far down the stream. A vault toilet stands near the camper parking area. You must bring your own water.

After setting up camp, check out the campground falls and pools. The waters of Jennings Creek plunge down the rocky face of a rhododendron-choked hollow into surprisingly large pools that invite a dip. Of course there are also trout in there. Licensed anglers can fish both up and downstream for small but scrappy rainbows. Upstream lies the Bald Mountain Ridge Scenic Area. This is my favorite hiking destination in the northern Cherokee National Forest. To explore the streams and hollows of Bald Ridge, pass through the campground archway and cruise up the wildflower-rich Jennings Creek Trail to the Little Jennings Creek Trail to reach Round Knob Picnic Area. Turn left onto the Cowbell Hollow Trail and pass through a rich forest to reach the Jennings Creek Trail. Return to camp and complete a 5-mile loop. A more ambitious loop continues from Round Knob Picnic Area up an old roadbed to reach the Appalachian Trail (AT). Turn left on the AT, straddling the state line to Jerry Cabin Trail shelter. Continue a bit farther to reach Coldsprings Bald, 4,500 feet in elevation. Here you will find a large field affording great views into Tennessee. Watch for the blue blazes to make the left onto the Sarvis Cove Trail. Descend steeply via many switchbacks, then come alongside Sarvis Creek, which has its own pools and cascades. The rhododendron can be thick down here. Reach the more open Poplar Cove Trail and make a left over a dry gap to get to Jennings Creek. Return down Jennings Creek to the camp for a 10-mile day. Less-experienced hikers should consider backtracking from Coldsprings Bald because the Sarvis Cove Trail can be rough and overgrown. Rest assured, a day hike in the Bald Mountains couldn't be nearly as rough as was a day for those who toiled at Old Forge as loggers. And they didn't return to such a pleasant setting along Jennings Creek as do tent campers today.

Old Forge Campground

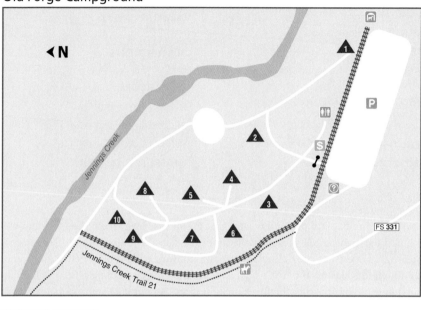

GETTING THERE

From I-26, take Exit 37 (TN 81/TN 107/Erwin/Jonesborough). Turn onto TN 107 West/TN 81 North, and drive 6.6 miles; then turn left to stay on TN 107 West, and drive 13.4 miles. Turn left onto Horse Creek Park Road, and drive 0.8 mile; then turn right to stay on Horse Creek Park Road, and drive 2 miles. Turn right onto Old Forge Road/Forest Service Road 331, and drive 2.5 miles to Old Forge Campground.

GPS COORDINATES N36° 05.409' W82° 40.923'

15

Paint Creek Campground

Beauty: ★★★★★ Privacy: ★★★★ Spaciousness: ★★★★★ Quiet: ★★★★ Security: ★★★ Cleanliness: ★★★★

Backing up to the Bald Mountains, Paint Creek is well situated for exploring the Greene County Highlands and historic Greeneville, the home of President Andrew Johnson.

The windshield wipers squeaked a decidedly unenthusiastic mantra the day we set out for Paint Creek. As we wound down the saturated road, the camping trip seemed more like a job than an outing. But our prospects brightened beyond the small bridge spanning Paint Creek. To our left lay the welcome sight of the Paint Creek Campground. Well laid out on an inside bend of Paint Creek, this cozy campground blends with its surroundings so beautifully that you'll think it was just meant for tent camping. Each campsite is ideally situated among the trees of the forest and is outlined with wood timbers that hold freshly spread gravel, making for an attractive and well-drained site. Eleven of the sites are directly creekside, but there are no bad sites at this campground. They're all large and well separated from one another by thick stands of preserved eastern hemlock, with plenty of room to pitch a tent and spread out a carload of gear.

Bicyclers pedal past a waterfall near Paint Creek Campground.

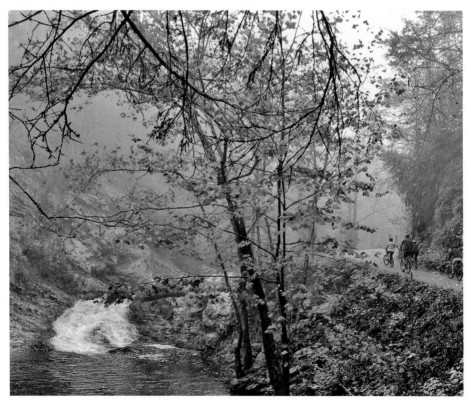

KEY INFORMATION

CONTACT: 423-638-4108, www.fs.usda.gov /cherokee

OPEN: Mid-May–October

SITES: 21

EACH SITE HAS: Fire grate, picnic table, lantern post, tent pad

ASSIGNMENT: First-come, first-served; no reservations

WHEELCHAIR ACCESS: Yes, 2 campsites

REGISTRATION: Self-register on-site

AMENITIES: Water spigots, vault toilets

PARKING: At campsites only

FEES: $10/night

ELEVATION: 1,640'

RESTRICTIONS:

PETS: On leash 6' or shorter

FIRES: In fire grates only

ALCOHOL: At campsites only

VEHICLES: Trailers up to 26'

OTHER: 14-day stay limit

Two small loops divide the campground. Vault toilets for each sex are unobtrusively placed on each loop. Water spigots are conveniently placed in the campground. There are no electric hookups. The northern loop has only six sites; half are along Paint Creek, a stream worthy of any mountain. The other 15 sites are on the southern loop, which follows Paint Creek as it descends toward the French Broad River.

The early spring sky cleared as we set up camp; the place was our own. After lunch we went for a drive along Forest Service Road 41, which parallels Paint Creek, to see Dudley Falls, which spills into a big pool backed by a rocky bluff. In warm weather, this pool is a popular swimming hole. The road bridges the creek and approaches smaller falls and fishing holes, meandering a 6 miles to Paint Creek's confluence with the French Broad River at Paint Rock. This road has become a popular bicycling destination too. The French Broad is a popular canoeing, kayaking and rafting river. Outfitters are stationed in Del Rio, Tennessee, and across the mountain in Hot Springs, North Carolina.

The Appalachian Trail (AT) is easily accessed from Paint Creek. Turn left out of the campground and head 5 miles up FS 31 to Hurricane Gap. The AT passes through the gap. Follow the AT to your right 0.8 mile up to the Rich Mountain Fire Tower, at an elevation of 3,643 feet. Look down on the French Broad Valley and gaze at the Bald Mountains around you. Mount Mitchell, the highest point east of the Mississippi River at 6,682 feet, stands tall to the east.

On our way home, we stopped in Greeneville, established in 1781. The citizens of this well-preserved town of old brick buildings have placed a special emphasis on keeping up the area's many historic sites, including the site of Civil War skirmishes and the home of President Andrew Johnson. Johnson's tenure as president was troubled, starting with his assuming the presidency after Abraham Lincoln's assassination and ending with his nearly being impeached by the Senate during Reconstruction. But the native sons of Greeneville are proud of their president. The National Park Service maintains a visitor center in Greeneville, and the town has undergone a revitalization and restoration of its historic downtown structures. Park your car and check out Johnson's home and tailor shop, the old churches, the Stone Jail, and the Harmony Cemetery.

Paint Creek Campground

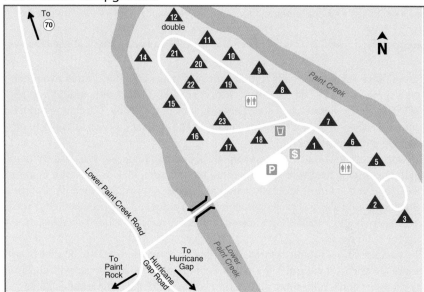

GETTING THERE

From Asheville, take I-26 North to Exit 19A (US 25 North/US 70 West/Marshall), and merge onto US 25 North. Drive 21.3 miles; then continue onto NC 208 North, and drive 3.5 miles. Turn left to stay on NC 208 North, and drive 5.6 miles. As you enter Tennessee, NC 208 North becomes TN 70 North; drive another 3.6 miles. Turn left onto Rollins Chapel Road, and drive 1.3 miles. Turn left onto Lower Paint Creek Road, and drive 1.7 miles (the pavement ends after 1.1 miles). Paint Creek Campground will be on your left after you cross the small bridge over Lower Paint Creek.

GPS COORDINATES N35° 58.669' W82° 50.674'

16

Pickett State Park Campground

Beauty: ★★★ Privacy: ★★★ Spaciousness: ★★★ Quiet: ★★★★ Security: ★★★★★ Cleanliness: ★★★★

Tennessee's first state park is a land of scenic geological and botanical wonders.

Tennessee State Parks come fully loaded with man-made amenities to help you make the most of your visit. But Pickett State Park was already fully loaded with natural features long before it became Tennessee's first state park way back in the 1930s. The campground is vintage too. It is evident that over the years Pickett's natural beauty, as well as the campground, have passed through caring hands.

The main camping area is situated atop a wooded hill. It has the standard circular loop configuration with a road bisecting the center of the loop, making almost a figure eight. You'll climb as you enter the loop. Most sites are on the outer edge of the loop, but the road that bisects the loop also has campsites along it. Tall pines and hardwoods shade the camping area. There is a light understory, mixed with more heavily wooded sections, especially outside the main loop.

The campground was built before RVs existed, so, even though 31 of 32 sites have both water and electricity, it is primarily a tenter's campground. A bathhouse with flush toilets and hot showers and a coin laundry are in the very center of the campground. Those staying on the campground's perimeter may have to walk a bit to reach the bathhouse. Speaking of walking, don't forget about the two walk-in tent sites.

The author's wife stands atop Pickett's Natural Bridge.

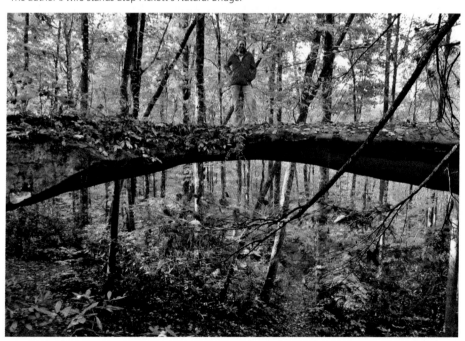

KEY INFORMATION

CONTACT: 931-879-5821,
  reserve.tnstateparks.com/pickett

OPEN: Year-round

SITES: 32, plus 2 walk-in tent campsites

EACH SITE HAS: Tent pad, fire grate,
  lantern post, picnic table, electricity

WHEELCHAIR ACCESS: None

ASSIGNMENT: First-come, first-served and
  by reservation

REGISTRATION: At visitor center

AMENITIES: Water, flush toilets, showers,
  laundry

PARKING: At campsites only

FEES: $15–$25/night, plus $5 reservation fee

ELEVATION: 1,500'

RESTRICTIONS:

PETS: On leash only

QUIET HOURS: 10 p.m.–6 a.m.

FIRES: In fire grates only

ALCOHOL: Prohibited

VEHICLES: None

OTHER: 14-day stay limit

Hand-laid stone walls complement the natural surroundings and blend in well with the campground. Even the park water tank is overlaid with stone. The campsites are a bit smaller than normal but offer more than adequate space. It's quiet and secure here in the outer reaches of Fentress County adjacent to the Kentucky state line. A park ranger lives on-site at the state park and the park visitor center is nearby.

You may need help figuring out just what to do. Recreational pursuits include tennis, badminton, horseshoes, and volleyball. Any equipment you may need is available free of charge at the park office. Before you imagine this is a wooded health club, let me assure you there's a lot more of the outdoor sort of fun, including a swimming beach open during the summer months at Arch Lake. This 15-acre, S-shaped lake offers trout fishing and canoe and rowboat rentals as well. Personal boats are allowed on the lake. A park naturalist is on duty during the summer. Headquarters are at the nature center, which is in the middle of the campground. Campfire programs and movies are also part of Pickett's activities.

Finally, and most importantly, there are the landforms, without which no man-made state park could exist. Much of the state forest escaped the logger's ax. Today, more than 58 miles of trails trace beneath the trees, reaching natural bridges, caves, waterfalls, and rock bluffs. The Indian Rockhouse Trail travels 0.2 mile to a huge rock overhang with a water feature in its center. The 2.5-mile Lake Trail Loop crosses Arch Lake on a swinging bridge then passes a natural bridge before looping back to the picnic area. It is 1 mile down to Double Falls from Thompson Overlook. Hazard Cave Loop extends 2.5 miles and goes by a sand-floored cave, then by the Natural Bridge, which is more than 80 feet long and 20 feet high.

The two primary park trails are Rock Creek and the Sheltowee Trace–Hidden Passage. The Sheltowee Trace Trail extends 280 miles into Kentucky. *Sheltowee* means "big turtle," which is what the American Indians called Daniel Boone way back when he was adopted into the Shawnee Tribe. The Rock Creek Trail parallels its namesake, passing small waterfalls in a classic, deeply wooded mountain stream. It is 5 miles one way and connects to the Sheltowee Trace Trail. Pickett's master trail is the Hidden Passage Trail, which runs in conjunction with the Sheltowee Trace. The first feature you'll see is a modest arch, then comes the Hidden Passage, a small passageway created by a large rock overhang amid jumbled rocks. Next is Crystal Falls, a delicate three-tiered watery drop. Continuing on down, you'll see overlooks and numerous rock houses, some with chestnut benches built by the Civilian Conservation Corps during the Depression. This rewarding loop continues after the Hidden Passage Trail diverges from the Sheltowee Trace. Any day hiking here will be a day you'll remember. Download a trail map from the park website. Recently opened and adjacent Pogue Creek Canyon State Natural Area adds another, wilder hiking dimension. This is one place where you can stay busy for days with all types of activities. Just make sure to get all your food and supplies back in Jamestown. You'll need the calories.

Pickett State Park Campground

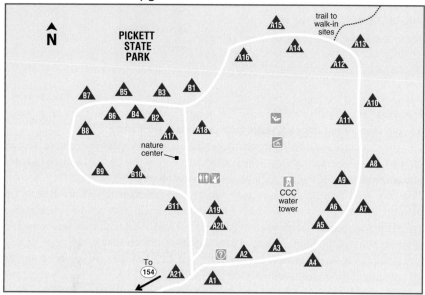

GETTING THERE

From I-40, take Exit 317 (US 127/Crossville/Jamestown). Turn onto US 127 North, and drive 33.9 miles (the last few will take you past Jamestown, on your left/west). Turn right on TN 154, and drive 12 miles; the park entrance will be on your left.

GPS COORDINATES N36° 33.101' W84° 47.888'

17

Rock Creek Campground

Beauty: ★★★★★ Privacy: ★★★★ Spaciousness: ★★★★ Quiet: ★★★★★ Security: ★★★★ Cleanliness: ★★★★

Camp in the cool and shady Rock Creek Campground adjacent to the impressive Unaka Mountain Wilderness.

Back in the 1930s, the Civilian Conservation Corps (CCC) developed the Rock Creek area for forest recreation, and Rock Creek Campground is one result of these Depression-era projects. As an antidote for an ailing economy, the CCC was assembled to provide jobs for unemployed men, although detractors of the organization accused the corps of doing "make-work." Here at Rock Creek (not to be confused with the Rock Creek on page 49), the CCC introduced the works of man into the wilds of East Tennessee to make the Cherokee National Forest more enjoyable for visitors. What a fine area they had to start with! The national forest is laden with virgin timberland and clear mountain streams that nestle against the backbone of the Unaka Mountains. Of course, the Forest Service has improved and maintained the area since the days of the Corps. But the old-time feel remains, as well as most of the original infrastructure. Today, as then, we can camp in the cool, shady cove of Rock Creek.

The campground is arranged in three loops. Mother Nature landscaped this place well, with tall hardwoods looming over a thick understory of moss, ferns, rhododendron, and small trees amid gray boulders. The farther back you go in the cove, the more this is evident.

Rock Creek Falls

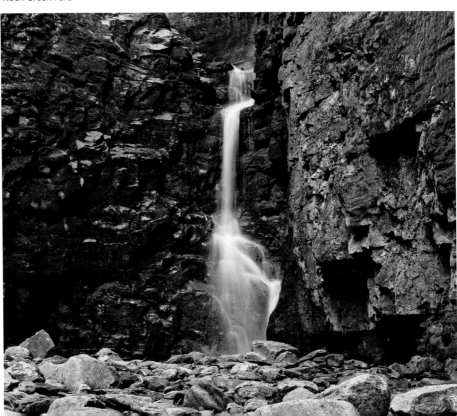

KEY INFORMATION

CONTACT: 423-735-1500, www.fs.usda.gov /cherokee; reservations: 877-444-6777, recreation.gov

OPEN: Mid-May–October

SITES: 33, plus 5 walk-in tent sites

EACH SITE HAS: Tent pad, lantern post, picnic table, fire pit, drive up sites also have electricity

WHEELCHAIR ACCESS: Some sites

ASSIGNMENT: First-come, first-served and by reservation

REGISTRATION: Self-register on-site

AMENITIES: Water, warm showers, flush toilets, swimming pool

PARKING: At campsites and walk-in lot

FEES: $20/night standard sites, $12/night walk-in tent sites

ELEVATION: 2,350'

RESTRICTIONS:

PETS: On leash only

QUIET HOURS: 10 p.m.–6 a.m.

FIRES: In fire rings only

ALCOHOL: Prohibited

VEHICLES: None

OTHER: 14-day stay limit

The white noise of Rock Creek is your constant companion here. Loop A has 10 sites, each with a parking area large enough to accommodate an RV. Two Loop A sites are for group camping. Loop B has 11 sites, including 3 double sites. Loops A and B both offer electrical hookups and share a modern bathhouse with flush toilets and warm showers. Loop C is located farthest back in the cove, against a steep hill. It has a very thick understory for maximum privacy. Its 12 sites are ideally suited for tent campers. Farther up from Loop C are five walk-in tent sites for those with an inclination for solitude. There are two campground hosts.

One of the most intriguing features of Rock Creek Recreation Area is the swimming pool. Another product of the CCC's efforts, the pool is a concrete-and-rock-lined basin of clear stream water, lying behind a small dam. A creek runs into the head of the pool, which is circled by a walkway. Trout will be swimming with you. The Rock Creek Trail parallels its namesake, passing small waterfalls in a classic, deeply wooded mountain stream. A bathhouse with changing rooms, restrooms, and showers for each sex are nearby. The day was a bit cool for a swim during our visit, but some hardy youngsters were splashing about and having a good time.

Maybe you should save your swim until after a scenic hike in the Unaka Mountain Wilderness that borders the campground. Leave your vehicle at the campsite and depart directly from the campground. Rattlesnake Ridge Trail (Forest Trail 26) climbs east 3 miles to the Pleasant Garden Overlook at 4,800 feet. At the base of Unaka Mountain is Rock Creek Falls. FT 26 leads out of the campground along the creek. A few creek crossings later, the falls' multiple descents come into view beneath the forest canopy—there is always something relaxing about a cascade. This hike to Rock Creek Falls is 2.3 miles one-way. Other short hikes leave from the campground. Take the 0.4-mile Hemlock Forest Trail Loop and find out about this important component of the Southern Appalachian woodlands. Then walk the 0.2-mile Trail of the Hardwoods Loop for comparison's sake.

Bicyclists have the 0.8-mile Rock Creek Bicycle Trail to enjoy as well. For any supplies you may need, Erwin is less than 4 miles away. However, it feels like civilization is light years away at Rock Creek Campground and the Unaka Wilderness.

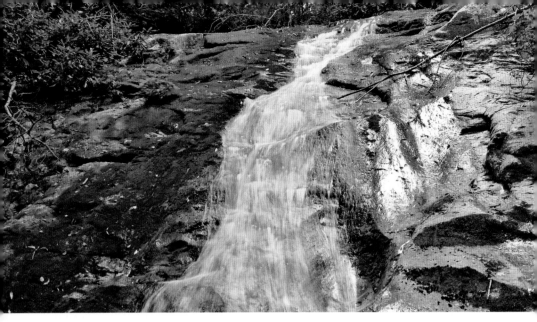

False Rock Creek Falls

Rock Creek Campground

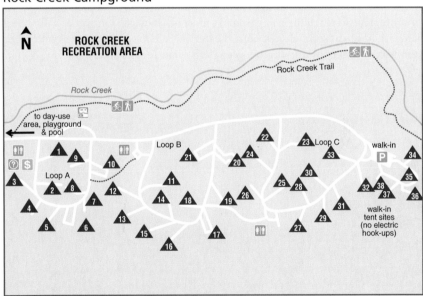

GETTING THERE

From I-26 near Erwin, take Exit 36 (Main Street/Erwin), and turn onto Harris Hollow Road (a right turn from I-26 West or a left turn from I-26 East). Drive about 0.3 mile; then turn right onto North Main Avenue, and drive 0.5 mile. Turn left onto TN 395 East, and drive 3.1 miles. Turn left into the Rock Creek Recreation Area; the campground will be on your right.

GPS COORDINATES N36° 08.263' W82° 20.947'

18

⚠ Round Mountain Campground

Beauty: ★★★★★ Privacy: ★★★★★ Spaciousness: ★★★ Quiet: ★★★★★ Security: ★★★ Cleanliness: ★★★

Enjoy the mountain meadow of Max Patch and lofty wooded camping.

Round Mountain Campground is off the beaten path in a seemingly forgotten corner of the Bald Mountains in Cherokee National Forest. Maybe it is the tortuously twisting gravel road that keeps most visitors away. We stayed here on a Friday night with good weather in mid-June, and only 3 of the 14 sites were occupied. The three other groups were tent campers. Those who find Round Mountain will relish the tranquil high-country campground that is so in tune with the woods that it seems to have been constructed by Mother Nature.

Round Mountain's sites are spaced along a single, thickly forested loop road that is bordered in moss—you are literally in the woods. Tall trees, including high-elevation species such as yellow birch and pin cherry, intermingle with white pine to provide a thick overhead canopy, shading all campers and the loop road. A junglelike growth of rhododendron on the forest floor separates the campsites. Noisy little streams cascade down the mountainside amid the brush.

The first two sites are actually picnic sites and are located on the approach road to the loop. The next five sites are placed among large trees and dense undergrowth. You must climb some steps to reach the campground's most isolated site. One other walk-up site is available. There are additional sites along the loop, where they blend in well with the scenery and feature plenty of distance between each other for maximum privacy. A comfort

Looking out from Max Patch

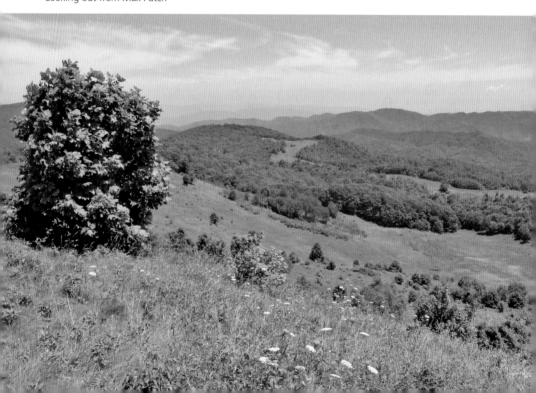

KEY INFORMATION

CONTACT: 423-638-4108, www.fs.usda.gov
/cherokee

OPEN: Late May–mid-October

SITES: 14

EACH SITE HAS: Tent pad, fire grate,
lantern post, picnic table, stand-up grill

WHEELCHAIR ACCESS: Yes, 1 campsite

ASSIGNMENT: First-come, first-served;
no reservations

REGISTRATION: Self-register on-site

AMENITIES: Vault toilets

PARKING: At campsites only

FEES: $7/night

ELEVATION: 3,100'

RESTRICTIONS:

PETS: On leash 6' or shorter

QUIET HOURS: 10 p.m.–6 a.m.

FIRES: In fire grates only

ALCOHOL: At campsites only

VEHICLES: 22' length limit

OTHER: 14-day stay limit

---

station with clean vault toilets for each sex is located at the loop's beginning. Make your last supply stop in Newport and don't plan on coming off Round Mountain until your stay is over. That winding road to and from civilization is a bear. Also, be certain to call ahead to verify that the campground is open if you plan to visit in early spring or late fall.

It's just a short distance from the campground to the Walnut Mountain Trail. Walk out to Forest Service Road 107, then go downhill 30 yards to reach the trailhead. It leads 1 mile to Rattlesnake Gap and another mile to the Appalachian Trail (AT) near the Walnut Mountain shelter. There will be attractive scenery regardless of which way you turn on the AT.

Our June journey took place on a cool mountain morning. Sunlight penetrated the forest canopy here and there, illuminating a light mist that rose from the woodland floor. The famed meadow that is Max Patch was waiting. We turned left out of the campground onto FS 107, motoring 2 miles up to Lemon Gap and the North Carolina border. The Appalachian Trail threads through these lovely groves, as it does in so many of the Southern Appalachians' treasure spots. On we drove, veering right at Lemon Gap onto FS 1182 and driving 3.5 miles farther, past a trout pond maintained by the Pisgah National Forest. Old-timers in overalls lounged in lawn chairs beside the pond, fishing poles in hand.

Beyond the pond, the forest opened to our left, revealing Max Patch in all its glory. The 230-acre field was once part of a working farm; the field now supports only wildflowers, which bloomed by the thousands, all facing the morning sun. We crested the top of the field at 4,629 feet and were rewarded with a 360° view. To the south stood the Great Smoky Mountains. Mount Sterling, with its metal fire tower, and Mount Cammerer, with its distinctive stone tower, stood out among the countless peaks. The open fields of the Bald Mountains stretched out to the north. It seemed as if we were in the very heart of the Southern Appalachians. We may have been.

Round Mountain is my favorite remote campground in this entire guidebook. Between the quiet solitude and classic, high-country atmosphere of each campsite, and the magnificence of Max Patch, this area exudes the best of the uplands that extend from the North Woods southward. It is hard to go wrong combining the beauty of the Appalachians and the charm of the South.

Round Mountain Campground

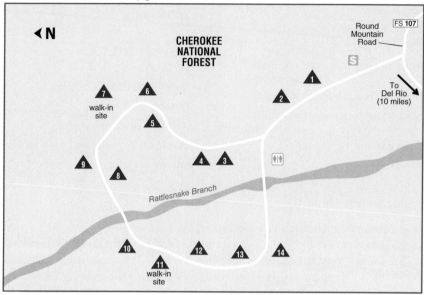

GETTING THERE

From I-40 West in North Carolina, take Exit 7 (Harmon Den). Turn right onto Cold Springs Creek Road, and drive 6.1 miles. Turn left onto NC 1182, and drive 0.2 mile; then turn left to stay on NC 1182, and drive 5.2 miles. As you enter Tennessee, NC 1182 becomes Round Mountain Road; drive 1.9 miles to the campground, on your right.

From I-40 East in Tennessee, take Exit 432B (US 25W East/US 70 East/Newport). Merge onto US 70 East, and drive 14.8 miles. Then turn right onto TN 107, and drive 6 miles. Turn left onto gravel FS 107/Round Mountain Road, and drive 5.9 miles to the campground, on your left.

GPS COORDINATES N35° 50.290' W82° 57.336'

NORTH CAROLINA CAMPGROUNDS

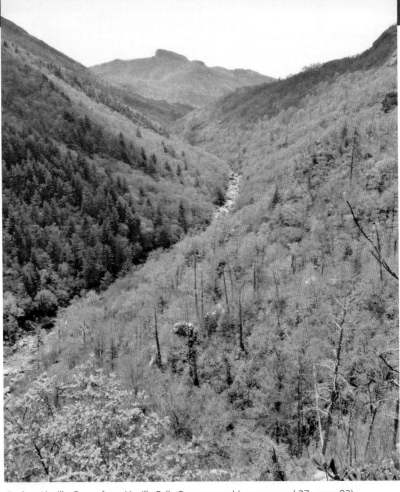

Explore Linville Gorge from Linville Falls Campground (campground 27, page 92).

19

Balsam Mountain Campground

Beauty: ★★★★ Privacy: ★★★ Spaciousness: ★★ Quiet: ★★★★ Security: ★★★★ Cleanliness: ★★★★

At 5,310 feet, Balsam Mountain is Great Smoky Mountains National Park's highest campground.

The rare spruce–fir forest that cloaks the highest elevations of the Smoky Mountains is among the primary reasons that this mountain range was designated as a national park. Covering 13,000 of the park's 500,000 acres, the forest composes the southern limit of this relic of the last ice age. More than 10,000 years ago, when glaciers covered much of the United States, woodlands much more reminiscent of those in Canada today migrated south. When the glaciers retreated, this forest survived on the highest points of the Smokies, creating an island of red spruce and Fraser fir trees.

So what does this have to do with tent camping? Well, it just so happens that Balsam Mountain Campground is located in a swath of this rare forest. Not only does it offer the highest tent camping within Great Smoky Mountains National Park, but it also offers campers a chance to experience this remarkable forest firsthand.

The campground was set up not long after the inception of the national park in 1934. Back then, few visitors drove or pulled oversize campers on the narrow, winding roads; the

View from the Flat Creek Trailhead

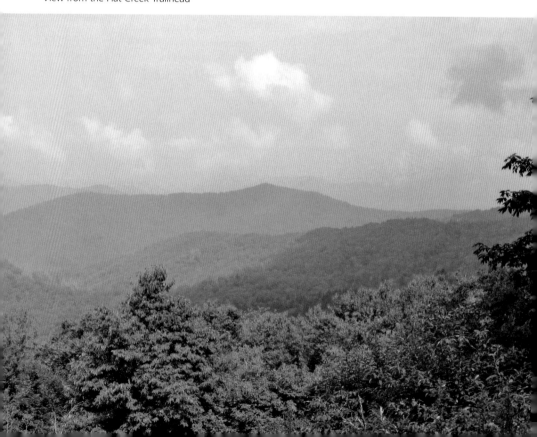

KEY INFORMATION

CONTACT: 865-436-1200, nps.gov/grsm;
reservations: 877-444-6777, recreation.gov

OPEN: Mid-May–early October

SITES: 45

EACH SITE HAS: Picnic table, fire grate

WHEELCHAIR ACCESS: Some sites

ASSIGNMENT: By reservation

REGISTRATION: Online

AMENITIES: Water spigot, flush toilet

PARKING: At campsites only, 2 vehicles/site

FEE: $17.50/night

ELEVATION: 5,310'

RESTRICTIONS:

PETS: On leash only

QUIET HOURS: 10 p.m.–6 a.m.

FIRES: In fire grates only

ALCOHOL: At campsites only

VEHICLES: 30' length limit

OTHER: 6 people/site; 14-day stay limit

majority tent camped. So when the campground was set up, builders had tent campers in mind. Today, we can camp in the fine tradition of the first park visitors.

Laid out in a classic loop, Balsam Mountain sits on a rib ridge between the headwaters of Flat and Bunches Creeks. Past the entrance station, campsites are set along the main road.

You will immediately notice the sites' small size, a historical element of Balsam Mountain that discourages most of today's RV campers. But even with the small sites relatively close together, you will find ample privacy because the campground rarely fills.

Keeping south on the main road, come to a loop. Campsites are spread along this loop among the fir and spruce trees. The ground slopes off steeply away from the road, resulting in some unlevel sites. With a little scouting, however, you will find a good site among the evergreens.

Balsam Mountain is off the beaten national park path. In fact, the road leading to the campground connects to the Blue Ridge Parkway, which then connects to the main body of the park. There is only one trail in the area, but it's a winner: Flat Creek. Leave the Heintooga Picnic Area on this path, and enjoy a magnificent view of the main Smokies crest before descending to the perched watershed of Flat Creek. Cruise through an attractive high-elevation forest before reaching the side trail to Flat Creek Falls, a steep and narrow cascade. Backtrack or continue past the falls to cross Bunches Creek and reach Balsam Mountain Road.

Balsam Mountain Road, just one of many interesting forest drives in the immediate area, leads 8 miles to the Blue Ridge Parkway, the granddaddy of all scenic roads in the Southern Appalachian Mountains, with recreation opportunities to both the north and south. A more rustic forest drive leaves Heintooga Picnic Area on a gravel road and runs north along Balsam Mountain before descending into Straight Fork valley to emerge at the nearby Qualla Cherokee Indian Reservation. There are several hiking trails along the way, including Palmer Creek Trail, which descends into a beautiful richly forested valley, and Hyatt Ridge Trail, which, along with Beech Gap Trail, makes for a rewarding high-country loop hike of 8 miles. Anglers can fish for trout on Straight Fork or enjoy many of the stream- and pond-fishing opportunities on the reservation. The nearby town of Cherokee has your typical Smokies tourist traps as well as camping supplies.

Balsam Mountain Campground

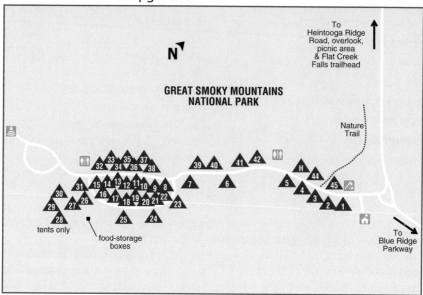

GETTING THERE

From I-40, take Exit 27 (US 74/US 19/Clyde/Waynesville), and merge onto US 74 West. Drive 3.7 miles; then take Exit 103 (US 19/Maggie Valley/Cherokee). Continue onto US 19 South/Dellwood Road, and drive 11.9 miles. Take the Blue Ridge Parkway exit on the right, and then turn left onto the Blue Ridge Parkway . Drive 2.4 miles; then turn right onto Heintooga Ridge Road, and drive 8.4 miles. Balsam Mountain Campground will be on your left.

GPS COORDINATES N35° 33.902' W83° 10.465'

20

Big Creek Campground

Beauty: ★★★★★ Privacy: ★★★ Spaciousness: ★★★★ Quiet: ★★★★★ Security: ★★★★ Cleanliness: ★★★★

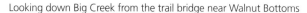

Only tents are allowed at this walk-in campground located in the Smokies' remote "Far East."

Great Smoky Mountains National Park has a reputation, somewhat undeserved, for being overcrowded. Sure, some places can become a bit peopled, but if you know the right places to go, your time in the park can be a relaxing getaway. Big Creek Campground is one of those places. It is the Smokies' smallest campground and its sole tent-only campground. This walk-in campground is set deep in the woods adjacent to the pure mountain waters of Big Creek—so deep, in fact, that when you come to the campground parking area, you'll wonder where the campground is. (For your information, it's between the campground parking area and noisy Big Creek.)

A small footpath leaves the parking area and loops the 12 campsites in the shade of tall hardwoods. Since Big Creek is a walk-in campground, you must tote your camping supplies anywhere from 100 to 300 feet. But after that, you'll be hearing only the intonations of Big Creek and smelling the wildflowers rather than hearing RV engines and smelling exhaust fumes.

Five of the sites are directly creekside. Each is spacious enough for you to spread out your gear. The new tent pads are elevated and well drained. A somewhat-sparse understory

Looking down Big Creek from the trail bridge near Walnut Bottoms

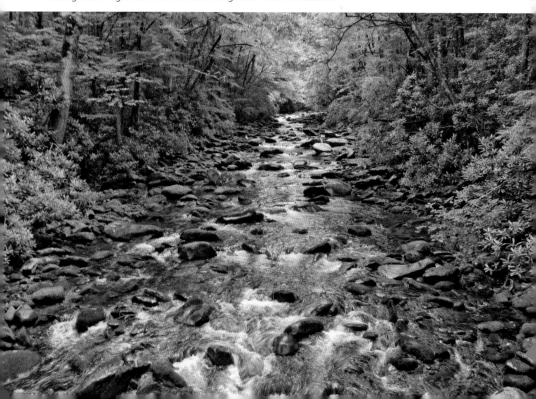

KEY INFORMATION

CONTACT: 865-436-1200, nps.gov/grsm; reservations: 877-444-6777, recreation.gov

OPEN: Mid-April–October

SITES: 12

EACH SITE HAS: Picnic table, fire pit, lantern post

WHEELCHAIR ACCESS: None

ASSIGNMENT: By reservation

REGISTRATION: Online

AMENITIES: Cold water, flush toilets

PARKING: At campsites only, 2 vehicles/site

FEE: $17.50/night

ELEVATION: 1,700'

RESTRICTIONS:

PETS: On leash only

QUIET HOURS: 10 p.m.–6 a.m.

FIRES: In fire pits only

ALCOHOL: At campsites only

VEHICLES: No RVs or trailers

OTHER: 6 people/site; 14-day stay limit

reduces privacy, but the intimate walk-in setup magnifies an atmosphere of camaraderie among fellow campers not necessarily found in larger drive-in campgrounds.

The campground comfort station borders the parking area. It houses flush toilets and a large sink with a cold-water faucet. Two other water spigots are found along the footpath loop. A recycling bin is located in the parking area.

You can explore the locale directly from your campsite. The Big Creek Trail starts at the campground and traces an old railroad grade from the logging era. Cool off the old-fashioned way in one of the many swimming holes that pool between the white rapids of Big Creek. Gaze up the sides of the valley; the rock bluffs you see have sheltered Smoky Mountain wayfarers for thousands of years. Hike two miles up Big Creek to find the tumbling cascades of Mouse Creek Falls. Falls often occur where a feeder creek enters a main stream; the primary stream valley erodes faster than the side stream valley, creating a hanging side canyon and then a waterfall. Continue on to Walnut Bottoms at 5 miles. Walnut Bottoms has historically had more man-bear encounters than anywhere in the park, so keep all food locked in your trunk, not in the seat of your car, when away from camp. Crestmont Logging Company had a camp here in the early 1900s, but now the area has returned to its former splendor. If you wish to explore further, three other trails splinter from Walnut Bottoms.

How about a strenuous hike through old-growth forest to a mountaintop capped by a Canadian-type forest with a 360° view from a fire tower? It's 6 steep miles up the Baxter Creek Trail, but your efforts will be amply rewarded. Start at the Big Creek picnic area just below the campground and go for it. Or take the Mount Sterling Trail from Mount Sterling Gap on nearby NC 284. It's only 2.7 miles to the tower this way. Alternately, hike the Chestnut Branch Trail, leaving from the Big Creek Ranger Station. It leads 2 miles to the highest and wildest section of the entire Appalachian Trail in the South, traversing the Smoky Mountains. The historic fire tower at Mount Cammerer is only 4 miles farther. Or loop back on the Appalachian Trail to Davenport Gap, and road-walk a short piece back to the campground.

Big Creek is wilderness tent camping at its best. The walk-in setting is your first step into the natural world of the Smokies. The rest of your adventure is limited only by your desire to explore the 500,000 acres in Big Creek Campground's backyard.

Big Creek Campground

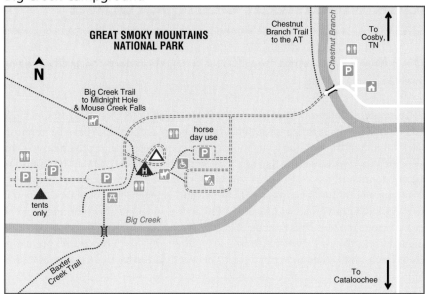

GETTING THERE

From I-40 in Tennessee, take Exit 451 (Waterville Road). From I-40 West, turn left onto Green Corner Road, and drive 0.3 miles; then turn left onto Tobes Creek Road. Or, from I-40 East, turn right onto Tobes Creek Road directly off the entrance ramp. Drive 0.1 mile over the Pigeon River; then follow the road as it immediately curves left and then right, becoming Waterville Road. Drive 2 miles; then continue onto Big Creek Road and into Great Smoky Mountains National Park. Drive 0.9 miles to Big Creek Campground.

GPS COORDINATES N35° 45.093' W83° 06.588'

21

Black Mountain Campground

Beauty: ★★★ Privacy: ★★★★ Spaciousness: ★★★★★ Quiet: ★★★ Security: ★★★★★ Cleanliness: ★★★★

The Black Mountain Recreation Area offers a family atmosphere and quality camping in a forested country setting.

Black Mountain Campground has been around for a long time. Over the years, it has been well maintained. Now it is like an antique, treasured by families that have been returning to Black Mountain through the generations. They come here to enjoy the relaxed country atmosphere in a forested setting that offers a sampling of the wild country in the shadow of the Black Mountains.

Cross the South Toe River on a wide bridge and enter Black Mountain Campground. To your right is a gravel road with a turnaround at the end. One of two campground hosts resides in a cottage there. This road parallels the Toe and contains 14 heavily wooded sites. Rhododendron shrouds these sites from one another. The six riverside sites are the most coveted. Two isolated sites are nestled far in the woods at the back of the turnaround.

Setrock Creek Falls is just a short walk away from the campground.

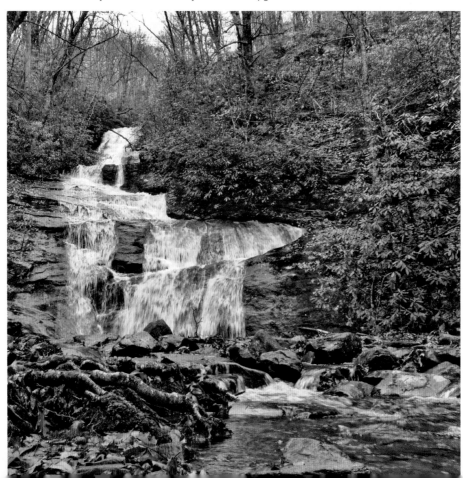

KEY INFORMATION

CONTACT: 828-682-6146, www.fs.usda.gov
/nfsnc; reservations: 877-444-6777,
recreation.gov

OPEN: April–October

SITES: 46

EACH SITE HAS: Tent pad, fire ring with
grill, picnic table, lantern post; 2 sites
have electricity

WHEELCHAIR ACCESS: Some sites

ASSIGNMENT: First-come, first-served
and by reservation

REGISTRATION: Self-register on-site

AMENITIES: Water, flush toilets

PARKING: At campsites only

FEES: $22/night, $29/night electric sites,
$44/night double sites (nonelectric)

ELEVATION: 3,200'

RESTRICTIONS:

PETS: On leash 6' or shorter

QUIET HOURS: 10 p.m.–6 a.m.

FIRES: In fire ring only

ALCOHOL: At campsites only

VEHICLES: 23' length limit

OTHER: 14-day stay limit June 1–September 1

Two water spigots are located along the road. A comfort station with flush toilets for each sex is situated midway along the road. A caged garbage disposal lies next to the comfort station. The garbage areas are caged because Black Mountain Campground once had a big problem with bears. Keep the Black Mountain bears wild and dispose of your trash properly. The main campground is on an oval road that loops a large field. There are 29 sites on this loop. The 12 sites on the interior of the loop by the field have more grassy understory beneath tall shade trees. Privacy is sacrificed for the openness of these sites.

The 17 sites on the exterior of the loop have a denser understory and are pressed against a hill, which required some site leveling. The tree canopy is thicker here, especially on the southwest side of the loop, where a small stream runs through rhododendron thickets. Two comfort stations lie at the farthest ends of the loop. Four water spigots make a cool drink easy to come by.

Three other sites are located along the road to the Briar Bottom Group Camp. They are close across the road from the Toe River and have a water spigot of their own. It is a bit of a walk to one of the three comfort stations, though. Sites 18 and 25 have electricity.

Children often play in the field at the main loop's center. A volleyball net was up on my weekday visit, yet the campground was very quiet. However, expect it to fill on summer weekends. Generally, tent campers constitute more than two-thirds of the patrons.

Adjacent to the main loop is the campground amphitheater. On weekend nights you can expect anything from local gospel groups to bluegrass pickers to ranger programs. The emphasis here is on old-fashioned family fun.

Bicycling, fishing, and hiking are the three most popular outdoor pursuits at Black Mountain Campground. Bring your bike and pedal the Briar Bottom Bicycle Trail. This trail starts at the Briar Bottom Group Campground, parallels the Toe River, and loops back around, crossing two bridges. It returns to the campground at 1 mile. From the Briar Bottom Bicycle Trail, you can take a foot trail a short piece to Setrock Creek Falls, a scenic cascade. Another moderate hike is the Devils Den Forest Walk. It begins at the main campground loop and makes a loop of its own during its half-hour woodland stroll.

For the strong-winded, the Green Knob Trail starts across the road from the campground and climbs 3.3 steep miles to a lookout tower at 5,070 feet. This is a strenuous hike. If you really want to check your physical condition, try the Mount Mitchell Trail. It starts near the amphitheater and climbs nearly 3,700 feet to the highest point east of the Mississippi.

The Toe River and its tributaries are well known for their trout fishing. But don't always expect to dip a line right by the campground on summer weekends. At that time, children are often swimming and tubing in the Toe's cool waters as it flows through the campground.

The setting and the activities are among the many reasons families and friends return to Black Mountain Campground again and again. Once you give it a try, you may come back here yourself.

Black Mountain Campground

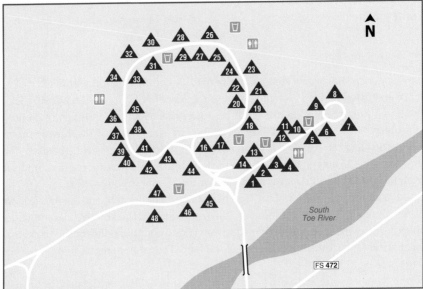

GETTING THERE

From I-40, take Exit 73 (Old Fort). Turn onto Catawba Avenue (a left turn from I-40 East or a right turn from I-40 West), and drive 0.5 miles. Turn right onto US 70 East, and drive 8.5 miles. Turn left onto NC 80 North, and drive 14.4 miles. Turn left onto South Toe River Road/Forest Service Road 472, and drive 3 miles to the campground, on the right.

GPS COORDINATES N 35° 45.115' W 82° 13.310'

22

Cable Cove Campground

Beauty: ★★★★ Privacy: ★★★ Spaciousness: ★★★★★ Quiet: ★★★★ Security: ★★★★ Cleanliness: ★★★★

Stay at Cable Cove and access the Smoky Mountains National Park by boat or land, free of traffic hassles.

Recent history is a theme of sorts for this charming and sedate campground, which sits on former farmland once tilled by the Cable family. After World War II began, the demand for aluminum and the power to manufacture it soared, leading to the construction of nearby Fontana Dam. Begun in 1942 and used to generate power to produce aluminum for the war, the dam remains an important source of energy. Prior to flooding behind the dam, the farming families moved away. The U.S. Forest Service moved in, later establishing a campground in the hollow.

Cable Cove's proximity to Fontana Lake makes it an ideal camp from which to visit the Smoky Mountains via boat, thus avoiding auto traffic. Fontana is a lightly used lake, with unlimited views of the park that are unspoiled by the troops of tourists that fill the highways on busy summer weekends.

Cable Cove Campground stretches out along a gravel road that slopes down toward Fontana Lake, a half-mile distant. A small loop at the end of the campground road enables drivers to turn around; this loop holds five campsites. Cable Creek, a small trout stream, parallels the road on the right. The campground is well maintained, quiet, and unassuming. Shortly after arriving, I felt as if I belonged there, like one of the neighbors.

Fontana Lake as seen from the Shuckstack Fire Tower

KEY INFORMATION

CONTACT: 828-479-6431,
www.fs.usda.gov/nfsnc

OPEN: April 1–October 31

SITES: 26

EACH SITE HAS: Tent pad, lantern post,
picnic table, fire grate

WHEELCHAIR ACCESS: Some sites

ASSIGNMENT: First-come, first-served;
no reservations

REGISTRATION: Self-register on-site

AMENITIES: Water, vault toilet

PARKING: At campsites only

FEES: $10

ELEVATION: 1,800'

RESTRICTIONS:

PETS: On leash only

QUIET HOURS: 10 a.m.–6 a.m.

FIRES: In fire grates only

ALCOHOL: At campsites only

VEHICLES: None

OTHER: 14-day stay limit

The 10 creekside sites are heavily wooded and have a thick understory. They are spacious yet have an air of privacy because of the junglelike vegetation along Cable Creek. The 11 sites opposite the creek have a grassy, gladelike understory beneath second-growth trees that are reclaiming the old fields. During my stay, the grass had been freshly trimmed and looked especially attractive. This "yard" space makes for a more open camping area, one conducive to visiting your neighbor, a customary thing to do in friendly western North Carolina. These campsites are some of the largest I have ever seen, extending far back from the road. An area of brush and trees divides the upper and lower campgrounds. Beyond the brush are the five sites at the turn-around loop, in the deep woods adjacent to Cable Creek.

Three water spigots have been placed at even intervals in the linear campground. Two comfort stations with flush toilets are at either end of the campground; campers in the middle may have to walk a bit to use them. But even this stroll could be an opportunity to get to know your neighbor. I camped toward the middle, and by the time I left, the gravel road resembled a country lane—slow moving and full of good friends.

Most of your fellow campers will be boaters. A high-quality boat ramp is a half-mile away; campers use it to fish for bream, bass, trout, and walleye, as well as to access the national park. (Using a boat to access the park is a smart way to beat the crowds. I've been doing it for over two decades and wonder why it hasn't caught on more.) Several hiking trails in the Smokies run right down to the lake. Check out the 360° view from Shuckstack Fire Tower. To reach the tower, which is visible from the lake, boat up the Eagle Creek arm of Fontana Lake. From the embayment, the Lost Cove Trail leads 3 miles up to the Appalachian Trail. Just 0.4 miles south on the Appalachian Trail is the tower. The outline of Fontana Lake is easily discerned from the tower. Look northeast and see the spine of the Smokies until it fades from view.

Across the water from Cable Cove is famed Hazel Creek, whose trout waters have been featured in fishing magazines for years. But don't visit just for the fish. Hike up the gentle trail that parallels the creek to discover relics of the Smokies' past, including old homesites, fields, and mining endeavors. Wide bridges spanning the creek make this walk even more pleasant. You can only access this part of the Smokies by boat or a very long walk; if you don't have a boat, contact Fontana Marina at 828-498-2129 to arrange for a shuttle.

The marina is only 4 miles west of Cable Cove. You can purchase limited supplies at the small store at Fontana Village Resort near the marina, but you're better off stocking up in Maryville, Tennessee, if you are coming from the Volunteer State, or in Robbinsville, North Carolina, south of Cable Cove on NC 143.

Also near Fontana Marina stands the engineering marvel that is Fontana Dam, the tallest dam east of the Rockies at 480 feet, and well worth a visit. A visitor center recounts the story of the dam, and cable cars take visitors down to its powerhouse. You can cross the dam in your auto—the landlubber's way to access the Smokies—at one of the more remote trailheads. From this trailhead, trace the Appalachian Trail 3.3 miles up to Shuckstack and its tower. Or take the undulating Lakeshore Trail through the Smokies' lush flora 5 miles to Eagle Creek and its embayment. Whether you get there by land or water, this slice of the Smokies is a gem to visit.

Cable Cove Campground

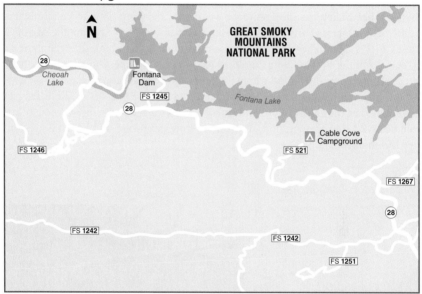

GETTING THERE

From I-40 in Knoxville, take Exit 386B (US 129/Alcoa Highway), merge onto US 129 South, and follow it 54 miles into North Carolina. Turn left onto NC 28 South, and drive 14 miles; then turn left onto Cable Cove Road, and follow it a short distance to dead-end at the campground.

GPS COORDINATES N35° 24.685' W83° 46.472'

23

Cataloochee Campground

Beauty: ★★★★★ Privacy: ★★★★ Spaciousness: ★★★★★ Quiet: ★★★★★ Security: ★★★★ Cleanliness: ★★★★

The Cataloochee Valley's remoteness and inaccessibility make it one of the Smokies' better-kept secrets.

Cataloochee Campground is only the first attractive spot you'll see in this valley of meadows, streams, mountains, history—and elk, which have been introduced into the valley and offer extraordinary wildlife viewing in Cataloochee's meadows. The celebrated fishing waters of Cataloochee Creek form one border of the campground, while a small feeder stream forms the other. In between is a flat, attractive camping area canopied with stately white pines. The attractions of Cataloochee Valley have increased the remote valley's popularity, resulting in advance reservations required for all campers in Cataloochee Campground.

Cataloochee Valley has ideal summer weather, with warm days and cool nights. An elevation of 2,600 feet is fairly high for a valley campground with a stream the size of Cataloochee Creek. Cataloochee uses the basic campground design: campsites splintering off a loop road. Six of the sites lie along Cataloochee Creek; a few others border the small feeder stream. All are roomy and placed where the pines allow. An erratic understory of hemlock and rhododendron leaves privacy to the luck of which site you draw. The campground host is situated at the entrance for your safety and convenience. Be forewarned: bears are sighted yearly at this campground, so properly store your food and keep the wild in the Smoky Mountain bears.

The Woody Place in Cataloochee Valley

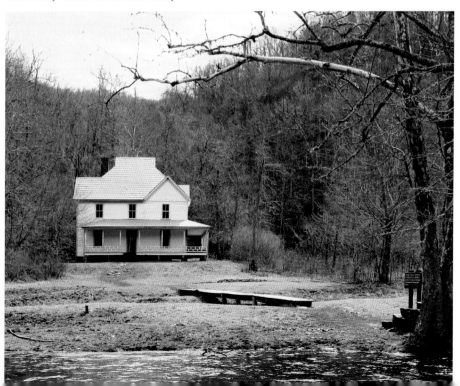

KEY INFORMATION

CONTACT: 865-436-1200, nps.gov/grsm;
reservations: 877-444-6777, recreation.gov

OPEN: Late-March–October

SITES: 27

EACH SITE HAS: Picnic table, fire pit,
lantern post

ASSIGNMENT: By reservation

WHEELCHAIR ACCESS: Some sites

REGISTRATION: Online before arrival

AMENITIES: Cold water, flush toilets

PARKING: At campsites only

FEE: $25/night

ELEVATION: 2,610'

RESTRICTIONS:

PETS: On leash only

QUIET HOURS: 10 p.m.–6 a.m.

FIRES: In fire pits only

ALCOHOL: At campsites only

VEHICLES: 31' length limit (not recommended for vehicles 25' or longer)

OTHER: 6 people/site; 14-day stay limit

Most RV campers shy away from this campground because the National Park Service advises against RVs making the long drive over rough gravel roads. Cataloochee fills up on summer weekends, yet with only 27 sites, it doesn't seem overly crowded. A comfort station is next to the campground at the head of the host. It has flush toilets and a cold-water faucet that pours into a large sink. Another water spigot is at the other end of the campground.

With all there is to do, you'll probably stay here only to rest from perusing the park. The first order of business is an auto tour of Cataloochee Valley. To gain a feel for the area, get a copy of the handy park-service pamphlet at the Ranger Station. An old church, a school, and numerous homesites are a delight to explore. Informative displays further explain about life long ago in this part of the world.

Cataloochee Valley is a hiker's paradise. Take the Boogerman Trail 7.4 undulating miles through different vegetation zones. The trail, which begins and ends at Caldwell Fork Trail, loops among old-growth hemlocks and tulip trees. Old homesites add a touch of human history; numerous footbridges make exploring this watery mountain land fun and easy on the feet. Or take the Little Cataloochee Trail to Little Cataloochee Church. Set in the backwoods, the church was built in 1890 and is still used today. Other signs of man you'll see include a ramshackle cabin, chimneys, fence posts, and rock walls.

The Cataloochee Divide Trail starts at 4,000 feet and rambles along the ridgeline border that straddles the Maggie and Cataloochee Valleys. To the north is the rugged green expanse of the national park, and to the south are the developed areas along US 19. Grassy knolls along the way make good viewing and relaxing spots.

Using the Rough Fork, Caldwell Fork, and Fork Ridge Trails, you can make another loop, this one 9.3 miles. Pass the fields of the Woody Place; then climb Fork Ridge, descend to Caldwell Fork, and climb Fork Ridge yet again to experience the literal highs and lows of Appalachian hiking.

The meadows of Cataloochee Valley are an ideal setting for a picnic. Decide on your favorite view and lay down your blanket. Nearby shady streams will serenade you as you look up at the wooded ridges that line the valley. Elk, deer, and other critters feed at the edges of the fields, drawing in nature photographers. Dusk is an ideal time to see Cataloochee's wildlife.

During our last stay at this campground, summer weather had finally hit. The air had a lazy, hazy feel as we toured the valley's historic structures. I fished away the afternoon, catching and releasing a few rainbows downstream from the campground. After grilling hamburgers for supper, we walked up the Rough Fork Trail to the Woody Place. The homestead looked picturesque as the late-evening sunlight filtered through the nearby forest. As we came back to the trailhead, deer browsed in the Cataloochee meadow. We knew we had come to the right place. So will you

Cataloochee Campground

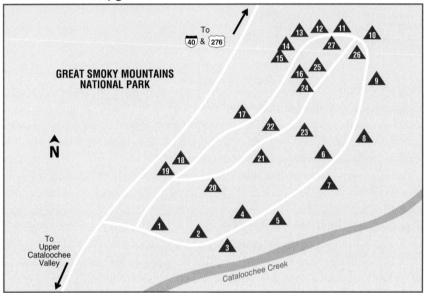

GETTING THERE

From I-40, take Exit 20 (US 276/Maggie Valley). Turn right onto US 276 South, and drive just 0.2 mile; then turn right onto Cove Creek Road/County Road 1395. Drive 5.7 miles to the entrance to Great Smoky Mountains National Park, and continue within the park for 1.8 miles. Turn left onto Cataloochee Entrance Road; then drive about 3 miles. The campground will be on your left.

GPS COORDINATES N35° 38.708' W83° 04.545'

24

⚲ Doughton Park Campground

Beauty: ★★★★ Privacy: ★★★ Spaciousness: ★★★ Quiet: ★★★ Security: ★★★★ Cleanliness: ★★★★★

Doughton Park Campground is much more than a way station along the Blue Ridge Parkway.

The National Park Service does a really good job with this Blue Ridge Parkway campground, which is located on the crest of the Blue Ridge and has a mountaintop ambience. A smart design spreads the campsites out and makes the area seem like several small campgrounds. Dividing the tent and RV sites into separate sections makes it even better. Twenty-one of the campsites can be reserved.

The 6,430-acre park and campground are named after U.S. Rep. Robert L. Doughton (1863–1954), a North Carolina Democrat who fought hard to help the parkway become the scenic reality it is. He would be proud of this area, which unobtrusively integrates modern structures into the historic dwellings and hiking trails that lace the park.

Before you explore Doughton Park, pick a campsite. This may take a few minutes, as the campground has several distinct areas. Open and airy, it is tastefully landscaped and well integrated into the ridgetop setting. Even the most discriminating tent campers will find a site to suit their tastes.

Views like this abound along North Carolina's Blue Ridge.

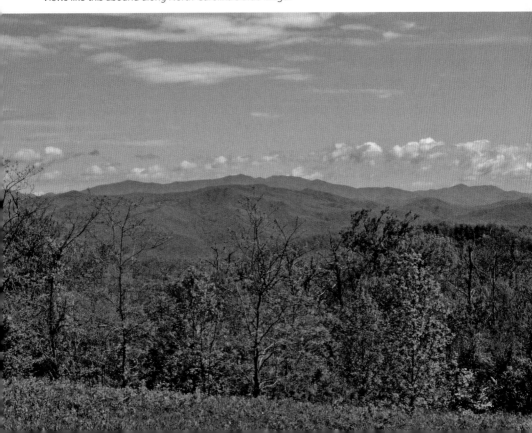

KEY INFORMATION

CONTACT: 828-298-0398, nps.gov/blri;
   reservations: 877-444-6777, recreation.gov

OPEN: Late-May–late October

SITES: 95

EACH SITE HAS: Tent pad, fire ring,
   picnic table

ASSIGNMENT: First-come, first-served and
   by reservation

WHEELCHAIR ACCESS: Some sites

REGISTRATION: At campground hut

AMENITIES: Water, flush toilets, pay phone

PARKING: At campsites only, 2 vehicles/site

FEES: $20–$35/night

ELEVATION: 3,600'

RESTRICTIONS:

PETS: On leash 6' or shorter

QUIET HOURS: 10 p.m.–6 a.m.

FIRES: In fire rings only

ALCOHOL: At campsites only

VEHICLES: None

OTHER: 6 campers/site, 30-day stay limit for
   calendar year

B and C Loops are for tent campers, and A Loop is reserved for RV campers. The first part of B Loop holds 22 sites and is heavily wooded, yet with a light understory. The sites undulate along a hill and are fairly close, so you may be a tad cozy with your neighbor. The comfort station is a ways down a sloping path, possibly a little farther than some are willing to walk.

Continuing along B Loop, sites 23–33 are set back in the woods, down from the paved campground road. Short paths lead back to them, so you will have to carry your gear to your site. This distance allows for the most rustic camping experience, out of sight from vehicles. The sites closest to the parking area border a grassy field adjacent to the parking area. Campers share the comfort station with the first loop via a short, paved path.

The rest of B Loop circles the highest point of the campground. It has 30 sites and is centered on a grassy glade where a water tank sits. Oddly enough, a campsite is located right by the water tank; when I checked it out, I found the view of the surrounding mountain lands worth the intrusion of the green structure. Other sites here offer intermittent views of the Blue Ridge and beyond. You even have a view from the comfort station at the loop's center. C Loop, directly west of B Loop, holds 31 additional tent sites.

The Blue Ridge Parkway is an exercise in scenic beauty, but I think this particular area is exceptional even for the BRP. A drive in either direction will sate your taste for dramatic landscapes and historic sites. The Brinegar Cabin is just a short distance north. Of course, the most rewarding views are those earned with a little sweat.

Doughton Park has more than 30 miles of trails that meander through pastures, along wooded ridges, and by mountain streams. The Bluff Mountain Trail departs from the campground and gives you a sampling of this country. It extends for 3 or so miles in each direction. The Fodderstack Trail, a 2-mile round trip, climbs to the Wildcat Rocks Overlook. Another recommended trail is Basin Creek, which ends at the Caudill Cabin (only accessible by foot). Cedar Ridge Trail begins at the Brinegar Cabin and drops down to Basin Creek. Before you hike any of these trails, though, download a trail map from the Parkway website. Then get out there and stretch your legs after enjoying that fantastic Blue Ridge Parkway scenery.

Doughton Park Campground

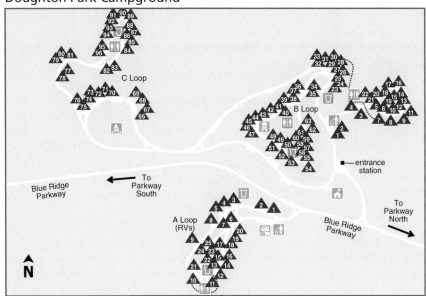

GETTING THERE

From I-77, take Exit 85 (NC 268 Bypass/Elkin). Turn onto NC 268 West, and drive 1.1 mile. Turn right onto the US 21 North ramp, and merge onto US 21 North. Drive 18.5 miles; then turn right at the sign for the ramp to the Blue Ridge Parkway. Turn right onto the Blue Ridge Parkway, and drive 9.8 miles. The campground will be on your right.

GPS COORDINATES N36° 25.733' W81° 09.266'

Brinegar Cabin at Doughton Park   *Photo: twbuckner/Flickr*

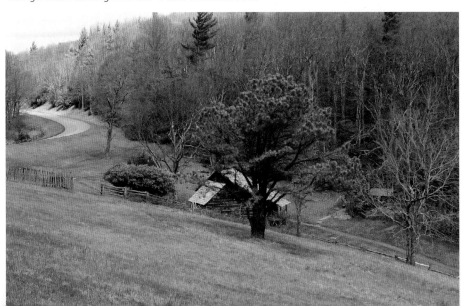

25

Horse Cove Campground

Beauty: ★★★★ Privacy: ★★★★ Spaciousness: ★★★★★ Quiet: ★★★★ Security: ★★★ Cleanliness: ★★★

Stay at Horse Cove Campground and enjoy the lovely trees of Joyce Kilmer Memorial Forest and the Slickrock Wilderness.

Horse Cove is an unpretentious, small campground adjacent to playful Lake Santeetlah (San-TEE-lah). Located primarily along Horse Cove Branch, a tributary of the lake, the campground with its minimal facilities has an unpolished, old-time feel. In a way, it is two campgrounds: the lower 6 being year-round sites and the upper 11 being warm-weather sites. The lower, year-round sites on Little Santeetlah Creek, another tributary, are across Forest Service Road 416 from the main campground and have a spur road of their own. A pit toilet is the only amenity, although water is available from a spigot in summer and from the creek in winter. These sites overlook the creek and lake from a heavily wooded knoll.

The upper campground runs up a narrow valley carved by Horse Cove Branch, which forms the western campground border. A steep mountainside hems in the campground to the east, but the campsites are graded and kept level with landscaping timbers; this hillside arrangement spreads sites apart both horizontally and vertically. A comfort station with a vault toilet is located at the campground entrance. And you're never far from one of the three water spigots that are conveniently placed about this cozy encampment.

A spare gravel road divides the upper campground. Beneath a hardwood canopy, the five sites beyond Horse Cove Branch are open and dry. They are well spaced along the road, which makes a short loop. The grassy center of the loop has a horseshoe pit. The six sites adjacent to boisterous Horse Cove Branch are isolated from each other by large rocks

The author admires the giants of Joyce Kilmer Memorial Forest.

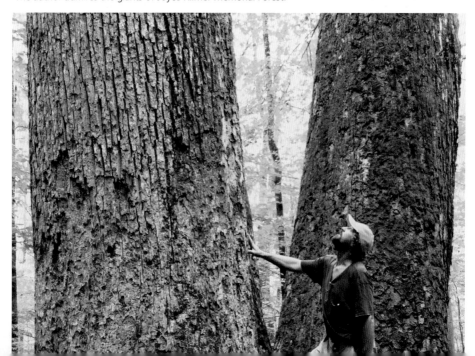

KEY INFORMATION

CONTACT: 828-479-6431, www.fs.usda.gov/nfsnc

OPEN: Upper campground, April 1–October 31; lower campground, year-round

SITES: 17

EACH SITE HAS: Tent pad, fire grate, picnic table, lantern post

ASSIGNMENT: First-come, first-served; no reservations

WHEELCHAIR ACCESS: Some sites

REGISTRATION: Self-register on-site

AMENITIES: Water in summer only, vault toilets

PARKING: At campsites only

FEES: $10/night April–October; $5/night in winter

ELEVATION: 2,300'

RESTRICTIONS:

PETS: On leash only

QUIET HOURS: 10 p.m.–6 a.m.

FIRES: In fire grates only

ALCOHOL: At campsites only

VEHICLES: None

OTHER: 14-day stay limit

intermingled with rhododendron and hemlock. The Horse Cove Trail leads to the high country right from the upper campground, then ends and splits into two trails along divergent railroad grades that remain from the logging days.

The reason for the campground's existence is its proximity to the magnificent Joyce Kilmer Memorial Forest and the adjoining Slickrock Wilderness. Hikers love to walk among the giants of this forest, named for the late writer Joyce Kilmer, who met an untimely end in France during World War I on July 30, 1918. Kilmer is best known for his poem "Trees," the first two lines of which are, "I think that I shall never see / A poem as lovely as a tree."

After Kilmer's death, a nationwide search ensued to locate a forest grand enough to memorialize him. Finally, a tract in North Carolina was selected. What we see today is a 3,800-acre, old-growth woodland that is one of the most impressive remnants of the Southern Appalachians before loggers permanently altered the landscape.

Several trails start at the Joyce Kilmer Memorial Forest parking area, which is 0.7 miles west of the Horse Cove Campground on FS 416. The Joyce Kilmer National Recreation Trail forms a figure eight as it loops through the forest. The 0.8-mile upper loop that travels through Poplar Cove is said to have the densest concentration of large trees in eastern North America. Tulip trees, 20 feet around the base, rise to meet the sun alongside their fellow forest dwellers: hemlock, beech, and oak. The largest cucumber tree in North Carolina is marked with a plaque.

You can't go wrong with any of the three trails that lead out of Joyce Kilmer Memorial Forest into the high country of the Joyce Kilmer–Slickrock Wilderness. A loop hike of differing combinations is possible using any of the Stratton Bald, Naked Ground, and Jenkins Meadow–Hangover Lead Trails.

For a scenic blockbuster of a hike, take the old Cherokee trading path, known to modern hikers as the Naked Ground Trail. It climbs 4.3 miles to Naked Ground, a spot named for its historical lack of trees. To your left it is 1.3 miles to Bob Stratton Bald, a mile-high mountain meadow with rewarding views of the Smokies and Nantahala National Forest. When cattle grazing ceased here, the field began to reforest. Later, trees were cut back and native grasses were planted. Consequently, the meadow and its beautiful views were restored. It's my favorite place in this wilderness.

From Naked Ground, it's 1.4 miles (right) to Hangover Lead. This sheer, rocky drop-off needs no assistance from the Forest Service to maintain its views. The Smoky Mountains and the open field of Gregory Bald are visible to your right. The lakes and mountains that are the legacy of western North Carolina and East Tennessee are all around you. Return via the Naked Ground or Hangover Lead Trail.

Horse Cove Campground

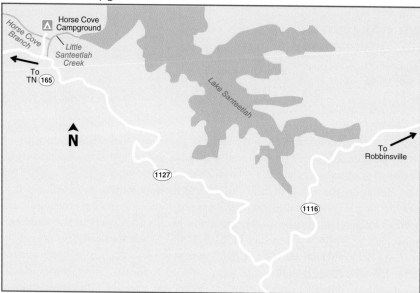

GETTING THERE

From I-75, take Exit 60 (TN 68/Sweetwater/Spring City), and turn onto TN 68 South. Drive 24.2 miles to Tellico Plains. Turn left onto TN 165 East/Cherohala Skyway/Unicoi Turnpike, and drive 41.6 miles. Turn left onto Santeetlah Road, and drive 2.4 miles to the campground.

GPS COORDINATES N35° 21.855' W83° 55.183'

26

Lake Powhatan Campground

Beauty: ★★★★ Privacy: ★★★★ Spaciousness: ★★★★ Quiet: ★★★★ Security: ★★★★★ Cleanliness: ★★★★★

This attractive, well-maintained mountain biker's heaven is on Asheville's doorstep.

Lake Powhatan is a nicely developed, well-maintained recreation destination. While it is a great destination in its own right, Lake Powhatan's proximity to Asheville adds the possibilities of visiting tourist destinations in the area, such as the grand Biltmore Estate. Hikers, mountain bikers, and lake enthusiasts will also find much to do at this Pisgah National Forest destination.

The groomed campground is divided into three loops situated on wooded hills above the lake. The Big John Loop has 21 sites—mostly shaded by a pine, oak, and hickory forest—and it is the highest of them all. Each site has been leveled with landscaping timbers, despite the hilliness. Large and attractive, the sites here provide ample privacy. The Bent Creek Loop has sites 22–35. It also has hilly, large camps with rich woods. All the sites here are in great condition. The Lakeside Loop, with sites 36–57, is actually well above Lake Powhatan, though a few of the sites overlook the water. The sites here are the shadiest, sheltered by hemlock trees.

The Hardtimes Loop, with sites 58–97, is my favorite. It's older than the others and looks a little more worn, yet is well kept. This least-used loop, set on a ridgeline rife with

Mountains frame Lake Powhatan. *Photo: Jennifer Pharr Davis*

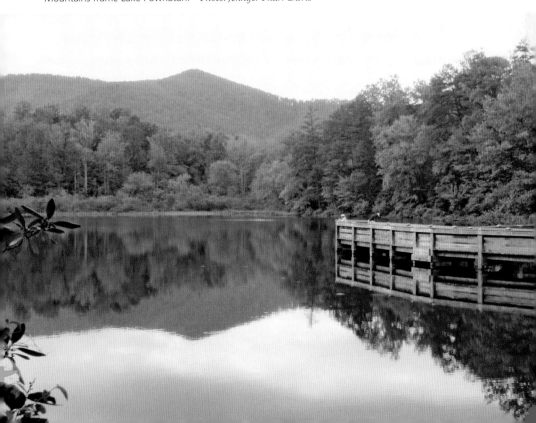

KEY INFORMATION

CONTACT: 828-670-5627, www.fs.usda
.gov/nfsnc; reservations: 877-444-6777,
recreation.gov

OPEN: March–October (Lakeside and
Big John Loops: March–December)

SITES: 97

EACH SITE HAS: Picnic table, fire ring,
lantern post; most sites have tent
pads; Lakeside Loop has electric, water,
and sewer

ASSIGNMENT: First-come, first-served and
by reservation

WHEELCHAIR ACCESS: Some sites

REGISTRATION: At entrance station

AMENITIES: Hot showers, flush toilets

PARKING: At campsites only, 2 vehicles/site

FEES: $22/night nonelectric, $28/night
electric

ELEVATION: 2,100'

RESTRICTIONS:

PETS: On leash only

QUIET HOURS: 10 p.m.–6 a.m.

FIRES: In fire rings only

ALCOHOL: At campsites only

VEHICLES: No length restrictions

OTHER: Reservations must be made 4 days
ahead of arrival and can be made up to
6 months in advance

---

dogwoods, actually has two loops. There are many attractive sites to choose from; you just have to be a little pickier. You will enjoy the pretty forest up here.

The campground is gated and manned with hosts who help keep the place in good, clean shape. Water spigots are conveniently set throughout. All the loops except Bent Creek have showers, but Bent Creek does have a restroom. Lake Powhatan can and does fill on summer holidays, but the reservation system will assure you of a campsite whenever you desire. Take advantage of it.

Bent Creek was dammed to form Lake Powhatan, an impoundment that is attractive to both swimmers and anglers. One side of the lake has a large beach and swimming area, while the other side has a fishing pier. The lake is stocked with rainbow, brook, and brown trout, and you can also fish Bent Creek. No boats are allowed on the lake.

A network of hiking and mountain biking trails weaves out from Lake Powhatan. The whole area is within the confines of the Bent Creek Research and Demonstration Forest. On the way in you will pass several national-forest mountain biking trailheads. Here you can make loops aplenty in the greater Bent Creek watershed, including up Wolf Creek, Ledford Branch, and Boyd Branch. Milder nature trails head directly out of the campground; one track circles the lake. The Deerfield Loop and Pine Tree Trail let you explore the woods without getting in your car. The former winds through a variety of ecosystems surrounding Lake Powhatan; the latter has interpretive information that helps you understand the forest through which you walk. The Homestead Loop is a short trail that passes over Lake Powhatan Dam. You do have to get in your car, but it is a short distance to visit the North Carolina Arboretum, which you will pass on your way in. Stop at the visitor center to learn more about this outdoor learning center.

Asheville is just a few miles up I-26; you'll find all manner of activities there.

The national forest offers interpretive programs between Memorial Day and Labor Day. Many of these are tailored to kids of all ages, so you can keep junior busy while you can get that much-needed R&R time.

Lake Powhatan Campground

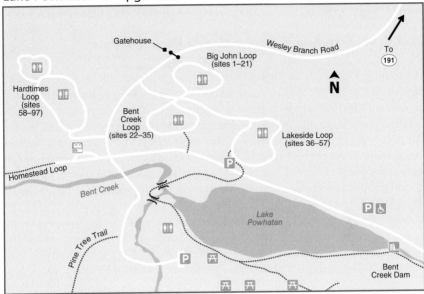

GETTING THERE

From the intersection of I-40 and I-26 in Asheville, take I-26 East, and drive 1.6 miles. Take Exit 33 (NC 191/Blue Ridge Parkway). Turn left onto NC 191 South, and drive 2 miles. Turn right onto Bent Creek Ranch Road, and drive 0.3 miles. Turn left onto Wesley Branch Road, and drive 2.1 miles. Stay left to stay on Wesley Branch Road, and drive 0.4 miles; then turn left toward the campground.

GPS COORDINATES N35° 29.010' W82° 37.512'

27

Linville Falls Campground

Beauty: ★★★ Privacy: ★★★ Spaciousness: ★★★★ Quiet: ★★★ Security: ★★★★★ Cleanliness: ★★★★★

Linville Falls lies at the head of the rugged Linville Gorge Wilderness.

The Blue Ridge Parkway is an unusual national park. It is linear, stretching 469 miles on the spine of the Southern Appalachians, connecting Great Smoky Mountains and Shenandoah National Parks. When deciding to designate the first national park in our Southern mountains, government officials just couldn't decide between Shenandoah and the Smokies, so both were developed. Because of this compromise, the scenic road connecting them was built. In the process, officials brought many historic sites and attractive natural features under the park-service umbrella. One of these outstanding areas is Linville Falls, the crown jewel of Linville Gorge, which many consider the most scenic wilderness in the Tar Heel State.

Linville Falls Campground, just off the parkway, can be your base for exploring the gorge. This campground is fairly large, with 70 sites, 50 of which are for tent campers. Oddly, the tent and trailer sites are intermixed along two paved camping loops with paved pull-ins. The setting, at 3,200 feet in elevation, is a flat alongside the clean, clear Linville River. A mixture

A hiker shoots a photo of Linville Falls.

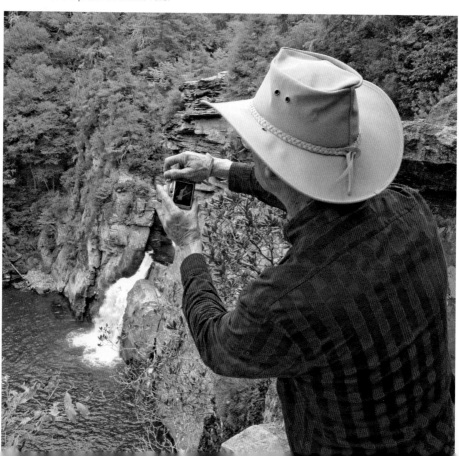

KEY INFORMATION

CONTACT: 704-298-0398, nps.gov/blri;
reservations: 877-444-6777, recreation.gov

OPEN: Mid-May–October

SITES: 50 tent-only, 20 RV

EACH SITE HAS: Picnic table, fire grate, grill

ASSIGNMENT: First-come, first-served and
by reservation

WHEELCHAIR ACCESS: Some sites

REGISTRATION: At campground
entrance booth

AMENITIES: Water spigot and flush toilets

PARKING: At campsites only, 2 vehicles/site

FEE: $20/night

ELEVATION: 3,200'

RESTRICTIONS:

PETS: On leash 6' or shorter

QUIET HOURS: 10 p.m.–6 a.m.

FIRES: In fire grates only

ALCOHOL: At campsites only

VEHICLES: 30' length limit

OTHER: 30-day stay limit for calendar year

of white pine, hardwoods, rhododendron, and open grassy areas allows campers to choose the amount of sun and shade they want. Along Loop A are several appealing tent sites set in the woods directly riverside.

On Loop B are two groupings of tent sites beneath beech trees. Your best bet is to cruise the loops and look for the site that most appeals to you. A sizable grassy meadow is free of campsites and makes for a great sunning or relaxing spot. The biggest drawback to the campground is its mixed placement of tent and trailer campsites. Nonetheless, choosy tent campers will be able to find a good spot. Water spigots are scattered about the campground, and the two bathroom facilities are located within easy walking distance of all the sites. For your safety and convenience, campground hosts and park personnel are on-site in the warm season. During winter, the water is turned off and vault toilets are used.

Linville Falls is your mandatory first destination. The falls, in two sections, drop at the point where the Linville River descends into its famous gorge. A park visitor center near the campground is your departure point. The Erwins View Trail is a 1.6-mile round trip that takes hikers by four overlooks, passing the upper and lower falls. The Upper Falls View comes first. You can see both falls from Chimney View. The Gorge View allows a look down into the deep swath cut by the Linville River as it descends between Linville Mountain and Jonas Ridge. Erwins View offers an even more expansive vista than the previous three. Another hike leads steeply from the visitor center down to the Plunge Basin, at the base of the falls. To access the main gorge, managed under the auspices of the U.S. Forest Service, campers must drive a short distance to Wisemans View Road and the Kistler Memorial Highway, a scenic auto destination rivaling the Blue Ridge Parkway. Below, the Linville Gorge Wilderness covers nearly 11,000 acres. Wisemans View is particularly scenic, allowing visitors to gaze up the gorge. Hikers have to trace steep and challenging trails to reach the river down in the gorge, and I know firsthand that they're pretty tough once you are in the gorge. A trail map of the gorge is available at the parkway visitor center. Bynum Bluff Trail makes a sharp drop down to a sharp bend in the river. Babel Tower Trail ends at a rock prominence encircled by the Linville River on three sides. Before taking off on any of these trails, you might want to get a hearty meal at the nearby Linville Falls community, where you can also buy limited camping supplies.

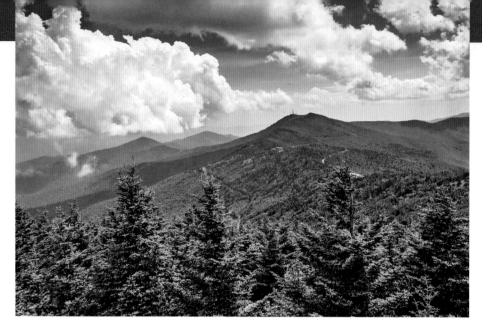

Linville Gorge in early autumn   *Photo: Craig Zerbe/Shutterstock*

Linville Falls Campground

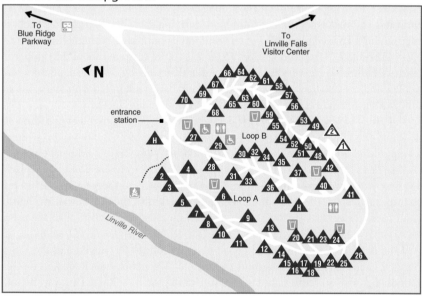

GETTING THERE

From I-40, take Exit 86 (NC 226/Marion/Shelby). Turn right onto NC 226 North, and drive 27.7 miles. Turn right at the exit for the Blue Ridge Parkway; then turn left onto the Blue Ridge Parkway. Drive 0.9 miles to the campground, on the right.

GPS COORDINATES N35° 58.368' W81° 56.148'

28

Mount Mitchell State Park Campground

Beauty: ★★★★★ Privacy: ★★★★ Spaciousness: ★★★ Quiet: ★★★★ Security: ★★★★★ Cleanliness: ★★★★★

The highest point in the eastern US is also home to its highest tent-only campground.

Bring warm clothes with you to Mount Mitchell—the rarefied air up here calls to mind Canada more than the South. The flora and fauna follow suit. In 1915, then–North Carolina Governor Locke Craig recognized the special character of this mountaintop and made it North Carolina's first state park. Now, with a tent-only campground and some superlative highland scenery, Mount Mitchell State Park is a Southern Appalachian highlight.

As the last ice age retreated north, cold-weather plants and animals of the north retreated with them, except for those that survived on the highest peaks down south. These mountaintops formed, in effect, cool-climate islands where the northern species continue to survive.

Mount Mitchell's campground is for tents only, unless you can carry an RV from the parking area up the stone steps to the campground. The short walk immediately enters the dense forest once dominated by the Fraser fir. Today, stunted and weather-beaten mountain ash and a few other hardwoods mingle with the firs.

The nine campsites splinter off the gravel path that rises with the mountainside. Set into the land amid the dense woods, they are small and fairly close together, but are private due to the heavy plant growth. There is little canopy overhead, as the trees become gnarled the higher they grow. Two water spigots lie along the short path; a bathroom with flush toilets is midway along the path. Firewood is sold by the bundle in the parking area.

Looking along the crest of the Black Mountains

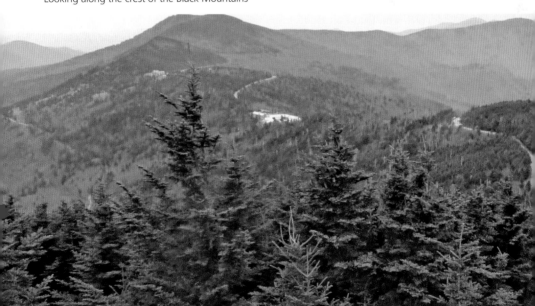

KEY INFORMATION

CONTACT: 828-675-4611; ncparks.gov
/mount-mitchell-state-park;
reservations: 877-722-6762,
reserveamerica.com

OPEN: May 1–October 31

SITES: 9

EACH SITE HAS: Tent pad, grill, picnic table

ASSIGNMENT: First-come, first-served and
by reservation

WHEELCHAIR ACCESS: None

REGISTRATION: Ranger will come by and
register you

AMENITIES: Water, flush toilets

PARKING: At designated parking area only

FEE: $17/night plus $3 online-reservation fee

ELEVATION: 6,320'

RESTRICTIONS:

PETS: On leash 6' or shorter

QUIET HOURS: 10 p.m.–6 a.m.

FIRES: In fire grates only

ALCOHOL: Not allowed

VEHICLES: None

OTHER: No gathering firewood in the park;
14-day stay limit

Sites 1 and 9 are the most private, but you'll feel lucky to get a site at all during summer weekends. This tiny campground exudes an intimate, secluded feel. The only noise you'll hear is the wind whipping over your head. By the way, Mount Mitchell is covered in fog, rain, or snow eight out of every ten days. Snow has been recorded every month of the year; 104 inches fall annually. Don't let those facts deter you, though—weather is part of the phenomenon that is Mount Mitchell.

The fog rolled in and out of the campground during our midsummer trip. Now and then the sun would shine, warming us. Wooded ridges came in and out of view with the fog; the whole scene seemed like some other world.

Carry a jacket along when you tramp the park. First drive up to the summit parking area, and make the short jaunt to the observation tower atop Mount Mitchell. Here lie the remains of Elisha Mitchell, who fell to his death from a waterfall after measuring the height of the mountain. From the tower you can see the Black Mountain Range and beyond. Back near the parking area, check out the museum that details the natural history of Mount Mitchell.

Many hiking trails thread the park. From the campground you can walk to the observation tower and connect to the Deep Gap Trail; it's a rugged 6-mile hike along the Black Mountain Range to several peaks that stand more than 6,000 feet high. Or you can leave the campground on the Old Mount Mitchell Trail past the park restaurant and loop around Mount Hallback to return to the campground.

Mount Mitchell State Park is surrounded by Pisgah National Forest, which is bisected by the Blue Ridge Parkway. This, in essence, increases the accessible forest area beyond the 1,860-acre state park. Many national-forest trails connect to the state-park trails, allowing nearly unlimited hiking opportunities. Procure a trail map from the park office for the best hiking experience.

Get your supplies in Asheville before you leave. Also check for the latest real-time road conditions on the Blue Ridge Parkway at nps.gov/blri. The Parkway makes for a scenic drive, but once in the highlands of the Black Mountains, you won't want to leave this wonderful mountaintop and campground.

Mount Mitchell State Park

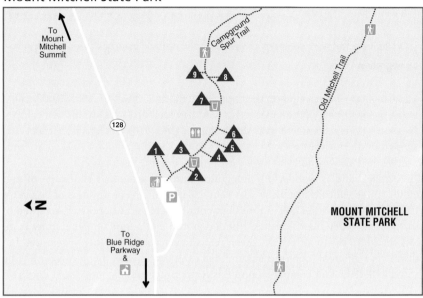

GETTING THERE

From Asheville, take I-240 East for about 4 miles, to where it becomes US 74 Alt East, and drive about 0.8 mile. Take the exit on the right toward the Blue Ridge Parkway, and from the ramp, turn right onto the Blue Ridge Parkway. Drive 29.4 miles; then turn left onto NC 128 into Mount Mitchell State Park. Drive about 3.4 miles to the campground.

GPS COORDINATES N35° 45.458' W82° 16.338'

An Appalachian vista from the Mount Mitchell observation tower   *Photo: John Bilous/Shutterstock*

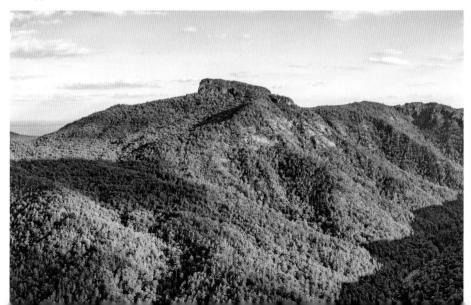

29

Mount Pisgah Campground

Beauty: ★★★★★ Privacy: ★★★★ Spaciousness: ★★★ Quiet: ★★★★ Security: ★★★★ Cleanliness: ★★★★

Loops exclusively for tent campers complement the natural beauty of this nearly mile-high campground.

This is the highest campground on the entire Blue Ridge Parkway at nearly 5,000 feet. And that is just the beginning of the superlatives here. Try secluded sites just for tent campers in a high-country forest, complete with stately spruce trees. How about nature trails circling the campground? Throw in some hot showers to the comfort stations. Add some fantastic views along the Parkway, and you have a great tent-camping destination.

The campground is wonderfully integrated into the mountain landscape of greater Mount Pisgah, specifically just below Flat Laurel Gap, amid the headwaters of Pisgah Creek and the 85-acre Flat Laurel bog, a rare high-country wetland where wind-sculpted birch and maple trees shade the campsites. Rhododendron and mountain laurel grow in dense thickets that offer plenty of privacy. Evergreens tower above all other vegetation. In this woodland, four different loops put like-minded campers together. Loop A is for RVs but is little used by RVs or tent campers. Loop B is for pop-ups and campers, so it doesn't have

The fire tower atop Frying Pan Mountain

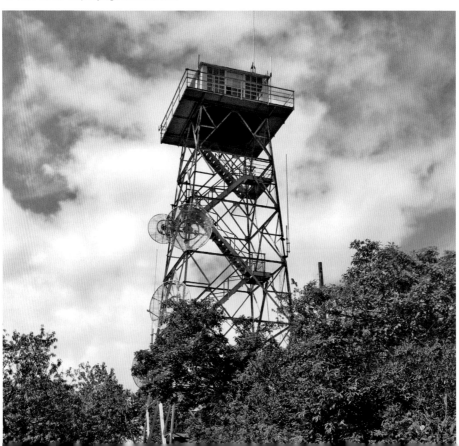

KEY INFORMATION

CONTACT: 828-298-0398, nps.gov/blri;
reservations: 877-444-6777, recreation.gov

OPEN: Mid-May–late October

SITES: 68 tent sites, 29 pop-up and van sites,
33 RV sites

EACH SITE HAS: Picnic table, fire
grate, lantern post; some sites have
tent pads

ASSIGNMENT: First-come, first-served and
by reservation

WHEELCHAIR ACCESS: Some sites

REGISTRATION: At campground kiosk

AMENITIES: Hot showers, flush toilets,
water spigots

PARKING: At campsites only, 2 vehicles/site

FEE: $20/night

ELEVATION: 4,980'

RESTRICTIONS:

PETS: On leash only

QUIET HOURS: 10 p.m.–6 a.m.

FIRES: In fire rings only

ALCOHOL: At campsites only

VEHICLES: 30' length limit

OTHER: 30-day stay limit for calendar year

tent pads, and the sites are less level than Loops C and D. Loop B has hot showers, as does Loop C.

Loops C and D are designated tent-camping loops, with 32 and 36 sites, respectively. Their tent sites are cut out of the forest, with heavy vegetation between them. Sometimes steps lead up or down to the sites from the paved auto pull-ins. If you have to look for a complaint, the sites are a tad small, and a few in C are a little close to the parkway. Overall, the sites are well maintained and well groomed, which adds to the already beautiful natural scenery.

Campsites are available without reservations any time except the major summer holiday weekends, but reservations can be made at any time. A campground host keeps things safe and orderly. Be apprised that food-storage regulations are in effect as a safeguard against bears. Because this campground is high, be prepared for cool conditions whenever you come. Bring a tarp to create a dry haven in case of rain.

The Blue Ridge Parkway sets the tone for Mount Pisgah, and you will enjoy great scenery on the way in. Once at the campground, you can enjoy walking some of the nature trails that form a network through and around the campground. Head to the tower atop Frying Pan Mountain or loop over to Buck Spring Gap; then walk to the top of Mount Pisgah, at 5,721 feet.

Not enough hiking opportunities? Why don't you visit Shining Rock Wilderness, just a few miles south on the Blue Ridge Parkway? I've enjoyed trekking here among the open fields, rock outcrops, and forests of this high-country preserve. Middle Prong Wilderness is less visited, more remote, and more wooded. Yellowstone Prong, a stream near Graveyard Fields Overlook south of the campground, has loop trails leading to three different falls, all relatively close together. The Cradle of Forestry Visitor Center is just a few miles down US 276 toward Brevard; see where the science of forestry began and explore some of the nature trails here. If you want to get wet, head down to Sliding Rock, a water feature on Looking Glass Creek where people shoot down a natural water slide into a pool. It's fun if you've never done it. Finally, the Mountains-to-Sea Trail traverses more miles along this area of the parkway than most hikers want to hike. A trail map of the Pisgah District of the Pisgah National Forest, which surrounds the parkway, comes in very handy here.

From the campground, a trail leads to the camp store, which sells some supplies and is near the Pisgah Inn on the other side of the parkway from Mount Pisgah. The inn serves breakfast, lunch, and dinner in case you don't feel like cooking. And you may be too tired to cook after all the hiking around here.

Mount Pisgah Campground

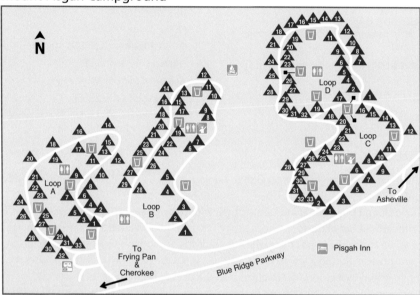

GETTING THERE

From the intersection of I-40 and I-26 in Asheville, take I-26 East, and drive 1.6 miles. Take Exit 33 (NC 191/Blue Ridge Parkway). Turn left onto NC 191 South, and drive 2.4 miles. Turn right onto the ramp to the Blue Ridge Parkway; then turn right onto the Blue Ridge Parkway itself. Drive 15.2 miles; the campground will be on your right.

GPS COORDINATES N35° 24.282' W82° 45.398'

30

Nelson's Nantahala Hideaway Campground

Beauty: ★★★ Privacy: ★★★ Spaciousness: ★★★★ Quiet: ★★★★ Security: ★★★★★ Cleanliness: ★★★★★

This campground offers easy access to the Nantahala River Gorge and numerous biking and hiking trails.

The owners of this facility knew they had a good location from which tent campers could access the numerous outdoor features in the immediate vicinity, so they set about creating a good campground to match the first-rate scenery of the area.

Pass the campground office, which has ice and soft-drink machines, and enter the campground. The design features the classic loop, which climbs up the side of a hill along a small creek, Powder Burnt Branch. The campsites are set along tiers that extend from one side of the loop to the other. This lets campers enjoy topographic relief without having to camp on a slope, as the tiers are level and evenly graded. The lower end of the loop is more open.

Several generations ago, the campground was a cornfield; later, trees reclaimed the site. When the campground was built, the many trees were left to flourish and naturally landscape Nelson's Hideaway. Tree cover thickens as the campground rises, with a thick carpet of grass forming the understory.

A section of the Bartram Trail in North Carolina

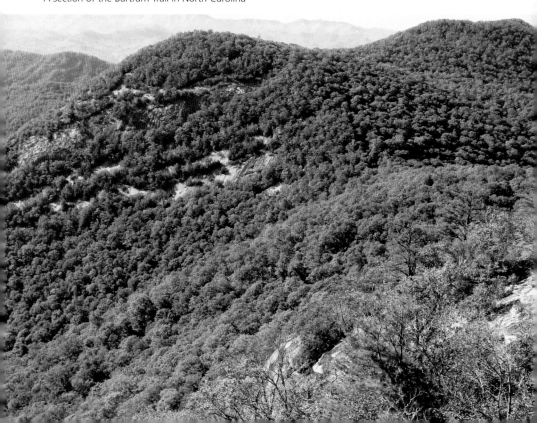

KEY INFORMATION

CONTACT: 800-936-6649 or 828-321-4407, nantahalacampground.com

OPEN: Mid-April–October

SITES: 43

EACH SITE HAS: Tent area, picnic table, fire ring

ASSIGNMENT: First-come, first-served and by reservation

WHEELCHAIR ACCESS: None

REGISTRATION: At campground office

AMENITIES: Water, hot showers, laundry, Wi-Fi, some electrical hookups

PARKING: At campsites only

FEES: $20/night; $30/night for 3 or more campers

ELEVATION: 2,800'

RESTRICTIONS:

PETS: On leash only

QUIET HOURS: None

FIRES: In fire rings only

ALCOHOL: At campsites only

VEHICLES: None

The centrally located bathhouse is simply the finest I've ever seen this side of a fancy hotel, much less a campground. Divided by sex, each attractive section contains three hot showers and flush toilets enclosed within a rustic wood exterior. Wash your dirty duds at the laundry facility, located here as well. Water spigots are spread throughout the campground.

If you don't feel like pitching a tent, use one of the Adirondack-style, open-air shelters at the beginning of the loop. They have padded bunks and a small porch where you can enjoy the cool mountain breezes. Each shelter has a picnic table beside it. They also offer cabins and a bunkhouse. Tent campers seek out the top of the loop, where the woods thicken and campers are kings of the hill. Here, you can see across the valley to the Snowbird Mountains.

The middle tiers are equipped with electricity in addition to the regular amenities. But don't expect too many RVs here: it's a steep climb to the campground from the highway. In addition, with all the hiking, canoeing, and kayaking opportunities, active campers are likely to be found here.

Just 2 miles north is a launch site for the Nantahala River Here, canoeists and kayakers enter the river gorge for a 9-mile run of nationally known whitewater floating. Commercial outfitters will accommodate inexperienced thrill seekers who long to challenge the chilly, continuous rapids.

The Nelson family has built hiking trails on its land that connect to the national-forest trails that border the campground. This is only fitting, as earlier family generations sold the land to the federal government to form a section of the Nantahala National Forest. The trails follow old routes that connected Cherokee lands in western North Carolina and eastern Tennessee.

The London Bald Trail is closest to the campground property. Reached from Piercy Creek, this trail connects to the Laurel Creek and Diamond Valley Trails, providing numerous loop-hiking opportunities. The Bartram Trail is also easily reached via the London Bald Trail. Consult the campground office or check their website for a collection of hiking maps.

Adjacent to the campground is a cool, clear fishing pond. An old-fashioned waterwheel oxygenates the water, in which trout thrive. For stream fishing, head to nearby Piercy Creek. Nantahala Lake is located just a few miles east for lake-fishing possibilities. An assortment of mountain biking trails threads the nearby national-forest land, which nearly envelops this campground.

Combine the fine facilities of Nelson's Nantahala Hideaway with the recreational variety of this section of western North Carolina, and you have a successful tent-camping adventure.

Nelson's Nantahala Hideaway Campground

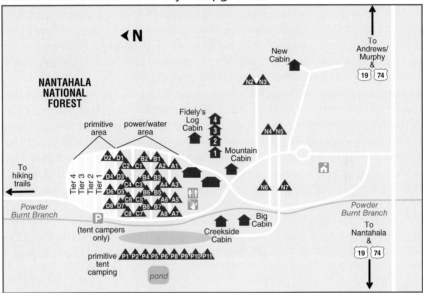

GETTING THERE

From I-75 near Cleveland in Tennessee, take Exit 25 (Cleveland/Dayton). Turn onto TN 60 South, and drive about 4.2 miles; then use the right lane to merge onto US 64 East (Ocoee). Drive 57.7 miles; then continue forward onto US 129 North/US 19 North/US 74 East, and drive 23.8 miles. The campground will be on your right.

GPS COORDINATES N35° 14.680' W83° 42.202'

31

North Mills River Campground

Beauty: ★★★ Privacy: ★★★★ Spaciousness: ★★★ Quiet: ★★★★ Security: ★★★★★ Cleanliness: ★★★★

This unhurried family campground rarely fills to capacity.

North Mills River Campground lies on the very edge of the Pisgah National Forest. But you would never know it by the sylvan setting of the area, divided by the free-flowing North Mills River, which has cut a valley amid the Carolina mountains. All roads leading to and within the campground are paved, which lures in a few extra RVers. Overall, this is an unhurried, family campground that is rarely filled to capacity.

As you approach the campground, it seems much larger than it really is, due to the sizable picnic area adjacent to the campground. To your right is a half-moon-shaped camping loop containing 13 campsites. These sites are in a very level area lying between the North Mills River and a steep hill. Tall shade trees grow high over the grassy understory. The five sites inside the half-moon are spread far apart and are mostly open. These sites are for the campers with excess gear who don't mind a slight sacrifice in privacy. Some sites on the outskirts of the loop are set into the hillside. The campground host resides on this loop. Four water spigots are evenly spaced among the campsites. A comfort station with flush toilets for each sex is at the loop's center.

The main campground loop is across a bridge over the North Mills River. These 12 sites are on a slight slope declining toward the river. As you drive along the one-way road, look

North Mills River

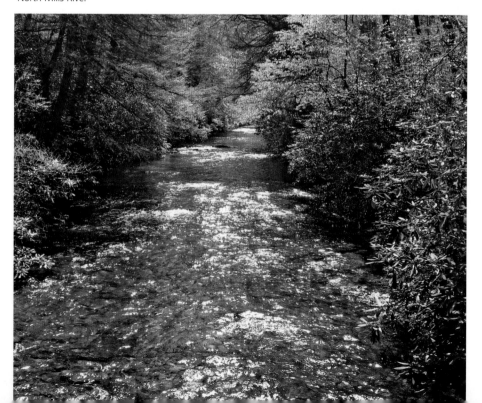

KEY INFORMATION

CONTACT: 828-877-3265, www.fs.usda
.gov/nfsnc; reservations: 877-444-6777,
recreation.gov

OPEN: Year-round; limited services
November–March

SITES: 26

EACH SITE HAS: Tent pad, picnic
table, fire ring; site 14 has full
hookups

ASSIGNMENT: First-come, first-served and
by reservation

WHEELCHAIR ACCESS: One site

REGISTRATION: Self-register on-site

AMENITIES: Hot showers, water spigot,
flush toilets, waterless toilet

PARKING: At campsites, 2 vehicles/site
($3/additional vehicle), and overflow lots

FEES: $22/night nonelectric, $31/night
full hookup

ELEVATION: 2,500'

RESTRICTIONS:

PETS: On leash only

FIRES: In fire grates only

ALCOHOL: At campsites only

VEHICLES: None

OTHER: 2 tents/site; 14-day stay limit

for a field inside of the loop. Four spacious and open sites are set in the field. A short spur road dead-ends off this loop and leads to three smaller campsites; this trio offers the most isolation in the entire campground.

As you continue along the main loop, the field gives way to an understory of hemlock, fern, and rhododendron growing amongst nearly hidden campsites. This understory grows very thick, especially as the loop parallels the river. Three single sites and one double site are located riverside beneath tall evergreens. Four water spigots are situated along the loop. A lighted bathroom lies in the dark and forested center of the loop.

North Mills River is used mostly by local families. Children float down the river in inner tubes, and anglers fish for trout, while others explore the nearby forest trails. As summer evenings darken and cool down, campers often meander from site to site and get to know their neighbors. Don't be surprised if you are paid a friendly visit and offered a cup of coffee by your fellow camper. The campground host is often the center of these social gatherings.

To get a good lay of the land combined with a little history, take a scenic forest drive. Gravel Forest Service Road 1206 leaves the campground just beyond the self-service pay station. It will lead you to the Pink Beds Visitor Center. The Pink Beds is a 6,800-acre mountain valley where professional forestry was first practiced in the United States. It is a National Historic Site complete with a museum that tells of the evolution of forestry in our country. Two interpretive trails enhance the story of George Vanderbilt's management of his forest-land. This valley is also known as the Cradle of Forestry in America.

To complete your scenic drive, turn right on US 276 from the Pink Beds and intersect the Blue Ridge Parkway after 3.8 miles. The Blue Ridge Parkway extends 469 miles, to link the Great Smoky Mountains and Shenandoah national parks. Head north on the parkway and enjoy some of the scenery for which this road is known. Stop and climb the 1-mile Frying Pan Mountain Trail to the lookout tower at its peak. Farther north is your right turn back onto gravel FS 479 and back down to the Mills River Recreation Area.

Informal hiking and fishing trails fan out from the campground. Several marked trails start 2 miles from the campground up FS 479 just after its junction with FS 142. The Big

Creek Trail (102) and Trace Ridge Trail (354) are two trails of note. They both leave the North Mills River watershed to intersect the Blue Ridge Parkway and the high country. If you're not sure exactly where to go, just ask your neighbor. Most local folks in the campground will gladly steer you onto a nearby good path. After all, they're quite proud of their mountain lands.

North Mills River Campground

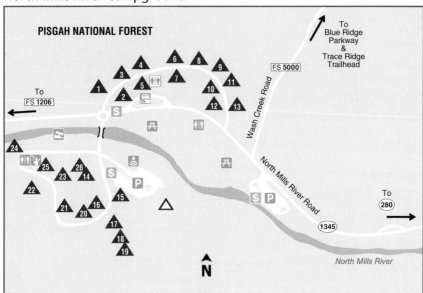

GETTING THERE

From I-26, take Exit 40 (NC 280/Asheville Regional Airport/Arden). Turn onto NC 280 West (a right turn from southbound I-26 or a left turn from northbound I-26). Drive 3.9 miles; then turn right onto North Mills River Road/NC 1345. Drive 5.1 miles to the campground.

GPS COORDINATES N35° 24.423' W82° 38.741'

32

Price Park Campground

Beauty: ★★★★★ Privacy: ★★★ Spaciousness: ★★★★ Quiet: ★★★★ Security: ★★★★ Cleanliness: ★★★★★

This campground is part of the Blue Ridge Parkway, yet it offers more than just a stopping place between scenic drives.

High in the forests of the Blue Ridge Mountains, Julian Price Memorial Park offers good camping and plenty of activities that don't involve an automobile. Don't let the size of the campground scare you off. There are nearly 200 sites in three areas: one area for RV camping only, one for one-night camping only, and another for both RV and tent camping.

The one-night-only camping loop backs against the shores of Price Lake. The south end of the paved loop is thickly forested, both overhead and on the ground, for maximum privacy. Five sites are right along the lakeshore. The other end of the loop circles a field and is more open. A few pull-through RV sites are here. A lighted bathroom is conveniently placed at the center of the loop for all campers to share. Two water spigots are located at each end of this spacious, private loop.

The main RV and tent area has three loops. Loops C and D spur off the larger Loop B. Oddly enough, Loop D is actually inside Loop B; Loop C spurs off on its own. All are in a rolling woodland and are set into the mountains without dominating the natural landscape. The plethora of trees overhead reminds you that you are in the forest. The

A summer afternoon along the Blue Ridge Parkway

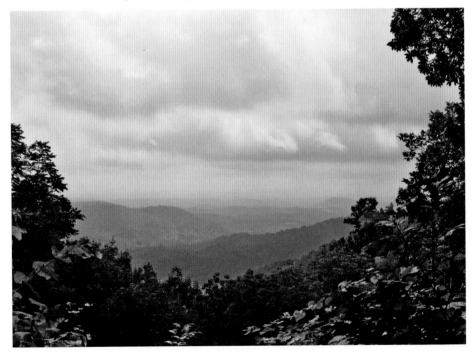

KEY INFORMATION

CONTACT: 828-298-0398, nps.gov/blri; reservations: 877-444-6777, recreation.gov

OPEN: Mid-May–late-October

SITES: 193

EACH SITE HAS: Tent pad, picnic table, fire grate, lantern post

ASSIGNMENT: First-come, first-served and by reservation

WHEELCHAIR ACCESS: Some sites

REGISTRATION: Register at campground check-in station

AMENITIES: Water, flush toilets

PARKING: At campsites only, 2 vehicles/site

FEE: $20/night

ELEVATION: 3,400'

RESTRICTIONS:

PETS: On leash 6' or shorter

QUIET HOURS: 10 p.m.–6 a.m.

FIRES: In fire grates only

ALCOHOL: At campsites only

VEHICLES: 30' length limit

OTHER: 30-day stay limit for calendar year

rhododendron understory provides plenty of privacy; however, it isn't everywhere, which means you can move about the campground freely. Landscaping timbers were used where site leveling was necessary. Some of the sites in Loops B and C are a tad close together, but with investigating and luck, you can find a private site. Prepare to search for the site you find desirable. Nine water spigots are scattered throughout these three loops for easy water access, and three lighted bathrooms ensure that you never have to go too far if nature calls in the middle of the night.

Loops E and F are for RVs only and concentrate these campers in one location. On my visit to Price Park, I didn't see any other RVers outside of E or F, with the exception of a couple in the one-night-only loop. Expect a full house on hot summer weekends, when nearby lowlanders escape the heat. However, I would take my chances on a first visit, to find a site you prefer in person, then note your favorite sites to make reservations on future visits. A ranger and a campground host reside at the campground to answer questions and ease your safety concerns.

Even the most ardent auto tourists have to stretch their legs every once in a while and see for themselves just what is beyond the roadside. Price Park offers the Blue Ridge sightseer plenty to do outside the car. Trails run through the campground, which makes starting a hike even easier.

The Boone Fork Trail makes a 5-mile loop passing through many environments of the Blue Ridge. It leaves the campground to enter a meadow and picks up an old farm road. It then runs along Bee Tree Creek, crossing it 16 times. Pass through a rocky area and return to the campground through a meadow.

The 2.3-mile Green Knob Trail climbs to an overlook that will reward you with well-earned views of Price Lake, then loops back via Sims Pond. The Tanawha Trail runs 13 miles south along the Blue Ridge Parkway and obviously requires a shuttle. A segment of the nearly complete North Carolina Mountains-to-Sea Trail passes through Price Park on its way to the Atlantic.

The Price Lake Trail makes a 2.3-mile loop around the 47-acre scenic tarn, which contains three species of trout that you can angle for: rainbow, brook, and brown. Nearby Sims Pond has only the native brook trout. Stream anglers can try Boone Fork and Sims Creek for trout as well. A valid North Carolina fishing license is required. Additionally, canoes and kayaks can be rented to paddle Price Lake.

During the 1940s, Julian Price bought this area as a retreat for his company employees. His heirs willed the area to the National Park Service for all of us to enjoy. As scenic as the Blue Ridge Parkway is, you may find this special area hard to pass. Stop and spend a day enjoying the sights without a windshield between you and nature.

Price Park Campground

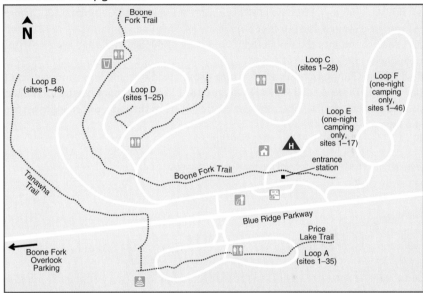

GETTING THERE

From I-40 near Marion, take Exit 86 (NC 226/Marion/Shelby). Turn onto NC 226 North, and drive 27 miles. Turn right onto NC 183 South, and drive 4.5 miles. Turn left to stay on NC 183 South, and drive 1.6 miles. Turn right onto the ramp toward the Blue Ridge Parkway; then turn left onto the Blue Ridge Parkway. Drive 15.9 miles to the campground, on your left.

GPS COORDINATES N36° 08.365' W81° 44.307'

Rocky Bluff Campground

Beauty: ★★★★ Privacy: ★★★ Spaciousness: ★★★ Quiet: ★★★★ Security: ★★★ Cleanliness: ★★★★

The design of this campground will capture your fancy, and the setting will make you stay.

As I headed down into the Rocky Bluff Recreation Area, I found it hard to believe that there was a campground there. The road dipped into hilly terrain, with nary a flat spot to be found. But soon enough, there was the beginning of Rocky Bluff Campground. *Engineering marvel* may be a stretch, but a ton or two of site leveling and stonework were necessary to fit this campground into the wooded dips and rises of the land. All that stonework makes your back ache just looking at it.

Rocky Bluff Campground is divided into two loops. Enter the lower loop as you pass the pay station. Three shaded sites are dug into the hillside and reinforced with the above-mentioned stonework. Five open sites sit on the inside of the loop, on what passes for flat ground here at Rocky Bluff.

Looking out from Lovers Leap toward the town of Hot Springs

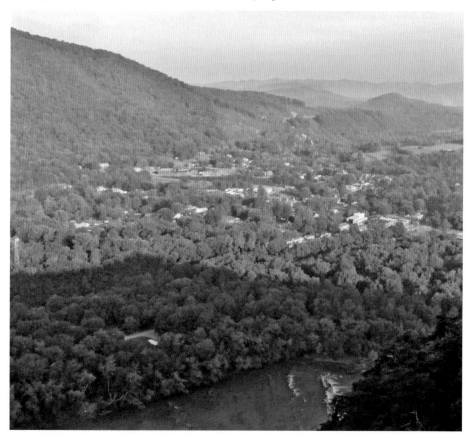

KEY INFORMATION

CONTACT: 828-689-9694,
www.fs.usda.gov/nfsnc

OPEN: Memorial Day weekend–
Labor Day weekend

SITES: 29

EACH SITE HAS: Tent pad, fire grate,
lantern post, picnic table

ASSIGNMENT: First-come, first-served;
no reservations

WHEELCHAIR ACCESS: Some sites

REGISTRATION: Self-register on-site

AMENITIES: Water, flush toilets

PARKING: At campsites only

FEE: $8/night

ELEVATION: 1,780'

RESTRICTIONS:

PETS: On leash 6' or shorter

QUIET HOURS: 10 p.m.–6 a.m.

FIRES: In fire grates only

ALCOHOL: At campsites only

VEHICLES: 18' length limit

OTHER: 14-day stay limit

At the low point of the lower loop, a road spurs off to the right and leads to the upper loop. As the road makes a steep climb, two campsites are somehow fit into the terrain. Seven sites lie on top of the hill, spread along the road as it makes a short loop to return to the main campground. Two sites offer a view into Spring Creek hollow to the east.

A warning to those who get spooked easily: also atop this hill, right next to the campsites, is Brooks Cemetery. Three sites look on to it. Stay down on the lower loop if the proximity of the cemetery will prevent you from enjoying a sound night's sleep.

Intersect the lower loop again from the upper-loop road. Here, sites are strewn in the open, lightly wooded center of the loop; a few more are tucked away in the thickets outside the loop. There isn't a whole lot of privacy. Due to the sloping terrain, you are probably going to be looking down on another camper or vice versa. A generally grassy understory doesn't shield you much from your neighbor, either. The upper loop, where ironically you might want to keep your neighbor in view to make sure he isn't a ghost roaming from the cemetery, is more wooded.

The lower-loop road passes a picnic area on the right and returns to the pay station. This loop has the only comfort station for the 29-site campground. Those on the upper loop must walk down the hill to use the facilities. But water spigots are conveniently placed around both loops for your convenience.

This campground is neat. The terrain and stonework make it unique, and the cemetery adds a touch of history and mystique. If the cemetery isn't enough of the past, imagine this place a century ago when there was a community of homes, a blacksmith shop, and a school.

The nearest community, Hot Springs, embodies small-town Appalachia. It's full of nice people who work hard for a living in the splendor of a land that is now more precious to them than ever before. The Appalachian Trail runs right through town. Visit the Pisgah National Forest Visitor Center, and check out the hot springs for which the community was named.

Outdoor pastimes are plentiful. Several outfitters in town will arrange a whitewater-rafting trip down the French Broad River, which flows through Hot Springs. A 6-mile biking trail runs along the river to Paint Rock, which marks the Tennessee–North Carolina state line. This dividing line crosses the bridge over the French Broad from Hot Springs. The Appalachian Trail crosses this bridge too. From here, make the short but rewarding climb to

Lovers Leap. Hike either way on the trail until your legs wear out. Then soothe your muscles in the actual hot springs, but you must pay for the privilege.

Two fulfilling trails depart from Rocky Bluff Campground. The 1.2-mile Spring Creek Nature Trail loops down to Spring Creek and follows it a good way before veering north and intersecting the campground again, making for a rewarding and short day hike. The Van Cliff Loop Trail is a little longer and tougher. It leaves the campground and climbs, crossing NC 209 on the way and hooking up into some piney woods before returning to the campground after 2.6 miles.

Rocky Bluff Campground

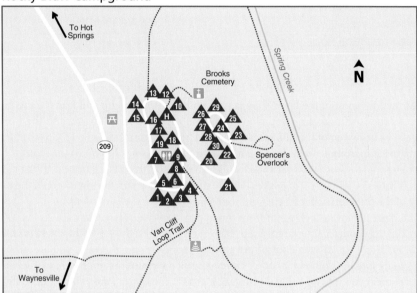

GETTING THERE

From I-26 near Weaverville, take Exit 19 (US 25 North/US 70 West/Marshall). From northbound, merge onto US 25 North/US 70 West; from southbound, turn right onto US 25 North/US 70 West. Drive 21.3 miles; then turn left to continue on US 25 North/US 70 West, and drive 5.1 miles. Continue straight onto NC 209 South/Lance Avenue, and drive 1.8 miles; the campground will be on your left.

GPS COORDINATES N35° 52.555' W82° 50.423'

34

Smokemont Campground

Beauty: ★★★★ Privacy: ★★ Spaciousness: ★★★ Quiet: ★★★ Security: ★★★★★ Cleanliness: ★★★★

Enjoy the North Carolina side of the Smokies while conveniently located near the town of Cherokee.

Smokemont is strategically located on the Oconaluftee River at the base of the Great Smoky Mountains. From this location, you can enjoy the immediate beauty of Great Smoky Mountains National Park and jump onto Newfound Gap Road northbound to explore other segments of the park. Take Newfound Gap Road just a few miles south, and you are in the tourist town of Cherokee. And if that isn't enough, you can take a ride on the Blue Ridge Parkway, which has just come 400-plus miles from Shenandoah National Park in Virginia to end near Smokemont. But this campground, nestled in a flat along Bradley Fork near the Oconaluftee River, exudes an old-time national-park camping atmosphere that may keep you mostly at your campsite, poking a stick into the fire, watching the trees grow, or listening to the water flow.

The campground is much longer than wide, stretching up the hollow of Bradley Fork, a fine, clear mountain stream that serenades the entire campground. Pass the ranger station and campground office. Campsites are strung out in loop form beneath the shade of oaks, maples, dogwoods, and hemlocks. The first loops, A and B, are open year-round, whereas C, D and F, the RV loops, may be closed in colder times.

Chasteen Creek cascades

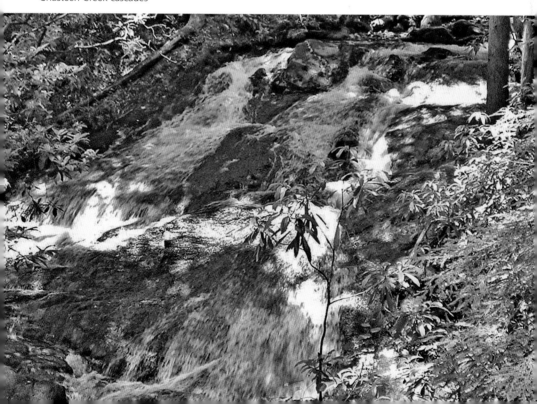

KEY INFORMATION

CONTACT: 865-436-1200, nps.gov/grsm;
reservations: 877-444-6777, recreation.gov

OPEN: Year-round

SITES: 96, plus 46 RV-only sites

EACH SITE HAS: Picnic table, fire grate,
lantern post; some sites also have
tent pads

ASSIGNMENT: First-come, first-served and by
reservation May 15–October 31

WHEELCHAIR ACCESS: Some sites

REGISTRATION: At entrance station

AMENITIES: Flush toilets, water spigots

PARKING: At campsites only, 2 vehicles/site

FEE: $21–$25/night, depending on season

ELEVATION: 2,200'

RESTRICTIONS:

PETS: On 6' leash or shorter

QUIET HOURS: 10 p.m.–6 a.m.

FIRES: In fire rings only

ALCOHOL: At campsites only

VEHICLES: 35' trailer length limit,
40' RV length limit

OTHER: 14-day stay limit

Overall, the sites are on the small side, and a lack of brush between campsites limits privacy. Strategically placed river boulders keep cars and campers separated. Old stone outbuildings house the bathrooms and also have outdoor sinks on them for washing dishes. Continue up the hollow to reach D Loop, which has more hemlocks. The sites are situated three wide here; the ones in the middle have less privacy. Shade is extensive throughout the campground and will be welcome in summer. Loop F is across Bradley Fork.

Summer is the busy time. Reservations are available between May 15 and October 31, so make them if you can. Campsites are available the rest of the year, and people do camp here year-round, even in the depths of winter. A word to the wise: store your food properly—this is bear country.

Simply being in the Smoky Mountains is the attraction. There is so much to see in the park. However, there is plenty to do right here in Smokemont, especially hiking. The Smokemont Loop Trail leads along Bradley Fork, then upward along the southern reaches of Richland Mountain and past the Bradley Cemetery, returning to the campground after 5 miles. The Bradley Fork Trail heads toward Cabin Flats, a backcountry campsite that makes a great day-hiking destination along upper Bradley Fork. If you are feeling aggressive, make a loop using Chasteen Creek Trail to see a waterfall then head to the high country along Hughes Ridge; then return via Bradley Fork, a good trout-fishing stream.

Speaking of fishing, here's a tip—the farther you get from the campground, the better the fishing. Oconaluftee River offers roadside trout angling. Or you can head up Big Cove Road or down into Cherokee for some ramped-up put-and-take fishing on Indian Reservation lands. The waters of the Smokies are not just for fishing, however. The cool streams are also good for a summer dip or even tubing. Be careful, though.

As previously mentioned, the Blue Ridge Parkway is good for an auto tour, or you can head up Newfound Gap Road and then onward to Clingmans Dome, the highest point in the park at 6,642 feet. It has a tower for observation. Stop for a visit at the park's Oconaluftee Visitor Center and see the pioneer buildings.

If you want a little touristy fun, head down to Cherokee, where you can buy some moccasins, get some taffy, or gamble at the reservation casino. If you're feeling cultural, check out the outdoor drama *Unto These Hills,* which is held nightly. Arts and crafts abound in town as well. For more info, visit cherokee-nc.com. Just remember you have some camping to do, too, at Smokemont.

Smokemont Campground

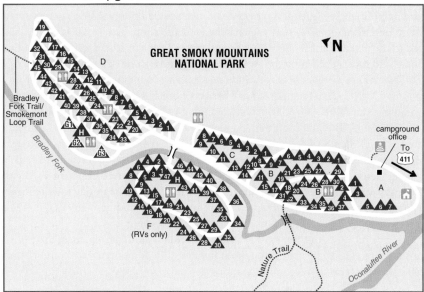

GETTING THERE

From I-40, take Exit 20 (US 276/Maggie Valley). Turn onto US 276 South, and drive 5.9 miles. Turn right onto US 19 South, and drive 20.4 miles. Turn right onto US 441 North, and drive 6.7 miles (you'll pass the Oconaluftee Visitor Center on your right). Turn right onto Smokemont Road, cross the river, and then immediately turn right, toward the campground.

GPS COORDINATES N35° 33.432' W83° 18.718'

35

Standing Indian Campground

Beauty: ★★★★★ Privacy: ★★★★ Spaciousness: ★★★★★ Quiet: ★★★ Security: ★★★★ Cleanliness: ★★★★

Soak in the mountains of the Standing Indian Basin from the headwaters of the Nantahala River.

According to Cherokee legend, a warrior was once posted on top of a certain mountain to look out for a flying monster that had snatched a child from a nearby village. The villagers prayed to the Great Spirit to annihilate the monster. A violent storm struck the mountain, reducing it to rock and turning the lookout warrior into a stone "standing Indian."

The Nantahala River is born on Standing Indian Mountain just upstream from this outstanding high-country campground, where cool breezes from the ridgetops temper the warm summer air. With sites on five loops, Standing Indian is spread out and offers a variety of site conditions. The first loop diffuses along the Nantahala with hemlock-shaded sites isolated by thick stands of rhododendron. Across the river, three loops are spread out in a large, flat area interspersed with large hardwoods that allow plenty of sun and grass to flourish among their ranks. Ritter Lumber Company once had a logging camp here. Farther back still, across Kimsey Creek, are mountainside sites. They stand level among the sloping forest of yellow birch, beech, and sugar maple, and are separated by lush greenery that makes each site seem isolated. Six double sites accommodate larger groups.

Campground hosts occupy each loop for your safety and convenience. Sixteen water pumps are strategically located throughout the loops, in addition to five comfort stations with flush toilets (two of the comfort stations also have hot showers). There are no electric

Big Laurel Falls is a great hiking destination for Standing Indian tent campers.

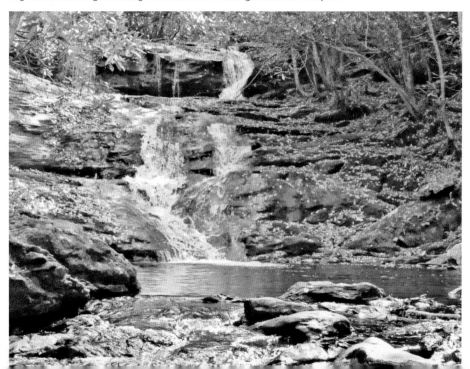

KEY INFORMATION

CONTACT: 828-524-6441, www.fs.usda
.gov/nfsnc; reservations: 877-444-6777,
recreation.gov

OPEN: April–October

SITES: 84

EACH SITE HAS: Tent pad, fire grate,
lantern post, picnic table

ASSIGNMENT: First-come, first-served and
by reservation

WHEELCHAIR ACCESS: Some sites

REGISTRATION: Self-register on-site

AMENITIES: Drinking water, flush toilets,
hot showers

PARKING: At campsites only

FEES: $16–$20/night

ELEVATION: 3,400'

RESTRICTIONS:

PETS: On leash only

QUIET HOURS: 10 p.m.–6 a.m.

FIRES: In fire grates only

ALCOHOL: At campsites only

VEHICLES: 21' length limit

OTHER: 14-day stay limit

hookups. You may pick up dead, downed firewood from the surrounding area without a permit. Keep in mind that Standing Indian can be crowded during peak summer weekends.

There's plenty to do nearby. Try your luck at one of the campground horseshoe pits. Fish for trout on the Nantahala River or Kimsey Creek. Rainbow and brown trout are the predominant cold-water fish in the streams, with some brook trout in the upper waters. For the nonfishing water lover, there are two falls nearby. Drive 5 miles on Forest Service Road 67 beyond the turnoff to the campground. The Big Laurel Falls Trail sign is on the right. After passing over a footbridge, the trail splits. Veer to the right and come to Big Laurel Falls in 0.5 miles. The Mooney Falls Trail starts 0.7 miles beyond the Big Laurel Falls trailhead and leads 0.1 mile to the cascading falls.

Several trails begin at the campground. To orient yourself, find the Backcountry Information Center 0.2 miles left of the campground entrance gate. Study the map. Make an 8-mile loop out of the Park Creek and Park Ridge Trails. The Park Creek Trail starts at the Backcountry Information Center; follow it down the Nantahala, then up Park Creek to Park Gap. Take the Park Ridge Trail 3.2 miles back down to the campground. This hike is moderate to strenuous, with a net elevation change of 880 feet.

The most prominent path in the area is the famed Appalachian Trail (AT), which skirts the campground to the south and east. The 87-mile section extending from the Georgia line to the Smokies is considered by many hikers to be one of the most rugged sections, with its relentlessly steep ups and downs. This section weeds out many thru-hikers who aspire to "follow the white blaze" 2,100 miles to Maine.

The AT passes FS 67 on the way to the campground. Drive out of the campground toward Wallace Gap about a mile. The Rock Gap parking area is on your right. Take the trail south (uphill to your right), and soon you'll come to the Rock Gap backcountry shelter, one of a series of shelters located about a day's walk from one another along the entirety of the trail. They provide a haven from the elements for the weary thru-hiker. Imagine this as your home for a six-month journey up the spine of the Appalachians.

While you're at Standing Indian Campground, why not see the mountain for which it was named? It's a strenuous 3.9-mile climb to the 5,499-foot peak, but the views provide ample reward. Use the Lower Ridge Trail, which starts on the left just beyond the campground bridge over the Nantahala. Switchback up to the ridge crest, and follow it southward to the AT. Take a spur trail 0.2 miles to the top of Standing Indian, and view the Blue Ridge Mountains and the Tallulah River Basin.

Standing Indian Campground

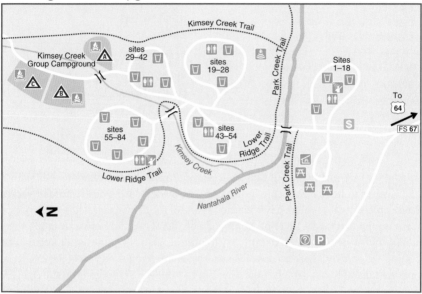

GETTING THERE

From I-75 near Cleveland in Tennessee, take Exit 25 (Cleveland/Dayton). Turn onto TN 60 South, and drive about 4.2 miles; then use the right lane to merge onto US 64 East (Ococee). Drive 57.7 miles; then turn right to stay on US 64 East, and drive 34.5 miles. Turn right onto West Old Murphy Road, and drive 1.9 miles to Wallace Gap. Turn right onto FS 67, and drive about 2 miles to the campground.

GPS COORDINATES N35° 04.328' W83° 31.850'

36

Tsali Campground

Beauty: ★★★★ Privacy: ★★★ Spaciousness: ★★★ Quiet: ★★ Security: ★★★★★ Cleanliness: ★★★★★

Head straight from the tent and go mountain biking, boating, horseback riding, hiking, or fishing.

What do a Cherokee, a pioneer, a big dam, and mountain biking have in common? Answer: They have all played a major part in the evolution of Tsali Recreation Area.

In 1838, during a forced removal of native peoples to the American West that became known as the Trail of Tears, a Cherokee leader by the name of Tsali turned himself in so other Cherokee could remain in the area. These natives formed the nucleus of the Eastern Band of Cherokee, who now live on a reservation adjacent to Bryson City. Early in this century, pioneer Harv Brown raised corn along Mouse Branch; there he turned his grain into "corn juice," otherwise known as moonshine. In the 1940s, when Fontana Dam was built, Harv and his kinfolk moved away. Now Harv's plot is Tsali Campground, where hikers, horseback riders, and especially mountain bikers congregate. These hearty adventurers catch their collective breath here at Tsali between excursions along the 39 miles of trails that emanate from the campground bordering Fontana Lake.

Tsali makes an ideal base camp for paddling Fontana Lake.

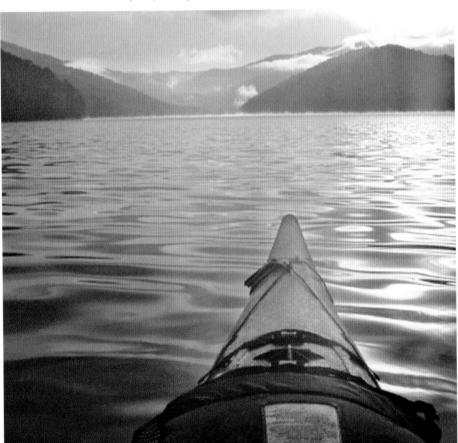

KEY INFORMATION

CONTACT: 828-479-6431,
www.fs.usda.gov/nfsnc

OPEN: April 14–October 31

SITES: 41

EACH SITE HAS: Tent pad, lantern post,
picnic table, fire grate

ASSIGNMENT: First-come, first-served;
no reservations

WHEELCHAIR ACCESS: Some sites

REGISTRATION: Self-register on-site

AMENITIES: Water, flush toilets, hot shower

PARKING: At campsites only

FEE: $15/night

ELEVATION: 1,750'

RESTRICTIONS:

PETS: On leash only

QUIET HOURS: 10 p.m.–6 a.m.

FIRES: In fire rings only

ALCOHOL: At campsites only

VEHICLES: None

OTHER: 14-day stay limit

Tsali Campground is divided into two loops, an upper and a lower. The upper loop has 22 sites. The U.S. Forest Service keeps the campground well groomed, and plenty of second-growth hardwoods and pines shade the former field. A sparse understory makes the campground open yet sacrifices privacy. Six of the sites are spread along Mouse Branch. Four water spigots are evenly dispersed along the loop. In its center sit a pair of low-volume flush toilets.

The lower loop features 19 sites and is more open and spacious than the upper loop, having fewer trees and, in some spots, a grassy understory. Eight sites back against Mouse Branch. At the head of the lower loop is a modern bath facility with flush toilets and hot showers, which are quite popular with sweaty hikers and bikers. Three water spigots are conveniently located on this loop, where a short trail leads down to Fontana Lake.

The campground is full on weekends and busy during the week with active campers. Mountain bikers from all over the Southeast converge on Tsali to ride its trails. Many campers bring kayaks as well, to drift on Fontana Lake and glide on the nearby whitewater rivers. Hikers abound; pleasure boaters and equestrians are represented, too.

There are four primary Tsali trails. The Forest Service has devised a system enabling hikers, bikers, and equestrians to enjoy the trails without bothering one another. Hikers can use all four trails at any time. The Right Loop and Left Loop Trails are paired, as are the Mouse Branch and Thompson Loop Trails, which are paired in a system whereby equestrians and bikers alternate using them daily. The Right Loop Trail is a singletrack trail that extends for 11 miles with views of Fontana Lake. It can be shortened to 4- or 8-mile loops. The Left Loop Trail is a 12-mile, singletrack pathway that features an overlook with a view of the Smoky Mountains. Mouse Branch Trail mixes a singletrack trail with old logging roads and passes through old homesites along its 6-mile course. You may see wildlife on the 8-mile Thompson Loop Trail, which crosses streams and passes through wildlife openings and old homesites. Check the trail-use schedule posted at the campground.

The boat ramp presents more recreational opportunities. You can fish in Fontana Lake or access the Smokies. Cross the water and anchor in any cove on the Smokies side of the lake. Then meander up the creek that created the cove, and you will run into the Lakeshore Trail, which runs for miles in both directions. Many relics of the past may be seen, including stone walls, chimneys, and broken china. Make it an adventure. But remember, all artifacts are part of the park and must be left behind for others to enjoy.

Other facilities at Tsali include a bike-washing area for cleaning up after those long, muddy rides; a stable for horses; and a bank-fishing trail near the boat launch for safely wetting a line. If you need supplies, drive west on NC 28 to Wolf Creek General Store.

This is a fun area for active people. Use Tsali as a base camp, and enjoy any and all of the activities available in this beautiful section of the Southern Appalachians.

Tsali Campground

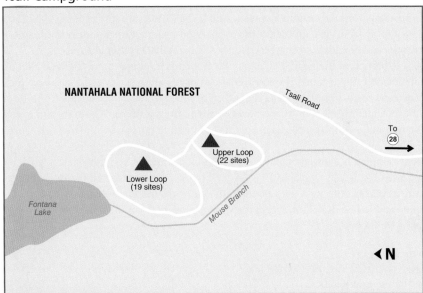

GETTING THERE

From I-40, take Exit 31 (US 74/US 19/US 23/Clyde/Waynesville). Merge onto US 74 West, and drive 48.5 miles. Turn right onto NC 28 North, and drive 3.5 miles. Turn right onto Tsali Road, and drive 1.5 miles; the campground will be on your left.

GPS COORDINATES N35° 24.355' W83° 35.195'

37

Van Hook Glade Campground

Beauty: ★★★ Privacy: ★★★ Spaciousness: ★★★ Quiet: ★★★ Security: ★★★★★ Cleanliness: ★★★★★

Van Hook Glade is strategically located near bucolic Cliffside Lake, the Cullasaja River and the town of Highlands.

The very name Van Hook Glade conjures up images of relaxing in an open field surrounded by forest. This image is only partly true. Van Hook Glade is a relaxing place, but now the area and campground are completely reforested. The 21 sites are spread along a single paved loop well away from one another, mostly separated by a mature woodland of maple, oak, white pine, and hemlock, so characteristic of the Nantahala National Forest.

A side branch of the nearby Cullasaja River wends its way around the west side of the mountainside campground. The individual campsites are well leveled. A few of the sites actually have a short series of steps that go up or down to the camping area from the road, lending an added touch of intimacy. Short, graveled trails lead from the loop road to a comfort station in the loop's center, where a hot shower and men's and women's flush toilets are available.

Tent camping is allowed at all the sites. Thirteen sites can accommodate a small RV or trailer. Sites are usually available on weekdays, but if you want Van Hook for the weekend, get a reservation. Although very popular, the campground is rarely noisy, with no group camping and so few sites. However, if the wind is blowing from the south, you can hear cars traveling on US 64.

The trees of Cliffside Lake reflect on still waters.

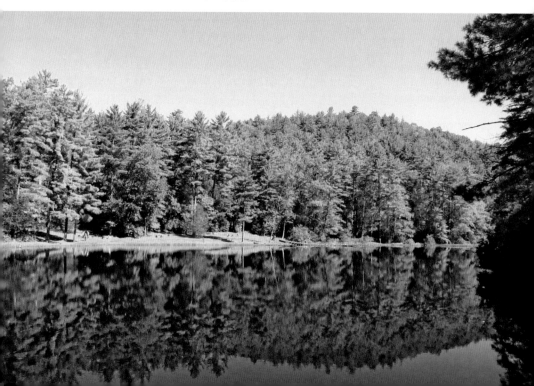

KEY INFORMATION

CONTACT: 828-526-5918, www.fs.usda
.gov/nfsnc; reservations: 877-444-6777,
recreation.gov

OPEN: April–October

SITES: 21

EACH SITE HAS: Tent pad, lantern post,
picnic table, fire grate

ASSIGNMENT: First-come, first-served and
by reservation

WHEELCHAIR ACCESS: Some sites

REGISTRATION: With campground host

AMENITIES: Water, flush toilets, hot shower

PARKING: At campsites only, 2 vehicles/site

FEE: $20/night

ELEVATION: 3,300'

RESTRICTIONS:

PETS: On leash only

QUIET HOURS: 10 p.m.–6 a.m.

FIRES: In fire rings only

ALCOHOL: At campsites only

VEHICLES: Not recommended for RVs

OTHER: 8 campers/site

Four miles of deep woods divide Van Hook Glade from the village of Highlands, over 4,000 feet in elevation. A short trip along US 64 will bring you to this highbrowed, summer community with restaurants, gift shops, and even a few places to get camping supplies. Highlands is the point of departure for the Mountain Waters Scenic Byway, a 60-mile drive that winds through the Nantahala National Forest to the town of Almond, near Fontana Lake. The byway follows US 64, old US 64, North Carolina 1310, and US 19.

Just out of Highlands you'll encounter the byway's first scenic feature, Bridal Veil Falls. You can actually drive your car under the 120-foot veil of water. Next, stop at Dry Falls. It's 3 miles west of Franklin. Take the 0.1-mile trail and descend to the falls. Then walk the trail that goes directly underneath the falls. You'll stay dry; that's how the falls got its name. West of Van Hook, US 64 winds precariously through the 7-mile Cullasaja Gorge to the town of Franklin. Near Franklin is 250-foot Cullasaja Falls. Drive with care, as there is no safe pullover at the cascading falls. (*Cullasaja* is Cherokee for "sweet water.") These are but some of the attractions on the Mountain Waters Scenic Byway.

The nearby Cliffside Lake Recreation Area provides plenty of nonmotorized activities for anyone staying at Van Hook. It is located 0.2 mile west of Van Hook Glade. Cliffside Lake is the result of the damming of Skitty Creek. Try your luck with some trout, swim the brisk mountain water at the beach, or take a hike. The 0.7-mile Cliffside Loop Trail crosses the dam while circling the four-acre lake. Start at the picnic parking lot and take the 1.5-mile Clifftop Vista Trail. You'll come to a gazebo from the 1930s at the cliff top; from there view the surrounding Cullasaja River country. Come back down the Clifftop Nature Trail. Helpful interpretive signs detail the flora of the area. Skitty Creek Trail leads down to US 64; it's an alternate route to Dry Falls. Take the 1.5-mile Homesite Road Trail down to US 64. You can walk 0.4 mile west to Dry Falls or 0.4 mile east to Bridal Veil Falls; either way, be careful on the road. Don't feel like driving at all? Take the 0.3-mile Van Hook Trail. It accesses the Cliffside Lake area in combination with a short hike on Forest Service Road 57. The Van Hook Trail starts between campsites 6 and 7 in the campground.

Between the town of Highlands and Cliffside Lake there's enough to keep anyone busy. And the Van Hook Glade Campground literally sits in the middle of it all in North Carolina's falls country.

Van Hook Glade Campground

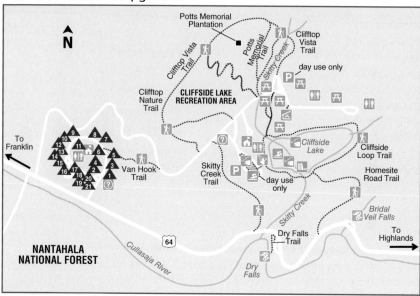

GETTING THERE

From I-40, take Exit 31 (US 74/US 19/US 23/Clyde/Waynesville). Merge onto US 74 West, and drive 26 miles. Take Exit 81 (US 23 South/US 441 South/Dillsboro/Franklin). Continue onto US 23 South, and drive 17.9 miles. Take the exit for US 64 East/Highlands/Franklin; then turn left onto US 64 East/NC 28 South, and drive 12.7 miles. The campground will be on your left.

GPS COORDINATES N35° 04.633' W83° 14.783'

SOUTH CAROLINA CAMPGROUNDS

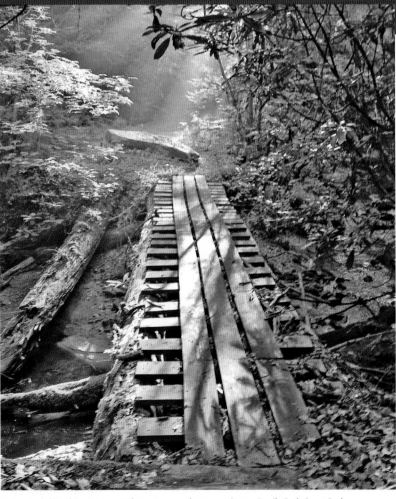

Enjoy trails like this one near Lake Jocassee when camping at Devils Fork State Park
(campground 40, page 132).

38

Burrells Ford Campground

Beauty: ★★★★ Privacy: ★★★★★ Spaciousness: ★★★★★ Quiet: ★★★ Security: ★★★ Cleanliness: ★★

The Chattooga River and Ellicott Rock Wilderness are just a few footsteps away from this primitive campground.

Before the Chattooga was declared a Wild and Scenic River, campers could drive all the way to Burrells Ford Campground. Since then, a protective river corridor has been established, effectively cutting off direct auto access to the campground. This has had mixed results: it has limited the use of the campground but has cut maintenance as well. The short walk may deter some tent campers, but you can guarantee that no RVs will ever be at Burrells Ford.

Follow the old jeep road down to the river, entering the protected corridor. The road forks at the river bottom, forested in tall white pines, with a thick understory of holly trees, rhododendrons, and mountain laurels. The Chattooga runs shallow and clear directly in front of the campground—no doubt the ford of days gone by. On the other side of the river lies the state of Georgia, deeply shaded in thick, junglelike vegetation. Deep pools lie both upstream and downstream of the campground, beckoning the camper to drop a line or take a dip. Rainbow and brown trout thrive in the mountain water.

The right fork of the old jeep road leads directly to the Chattooga. Campsites are spread along both sides of the road. Most are cooled beneath the shady canopy, but some lie in a

Johnny Molloy admires Kings Creek Falls.

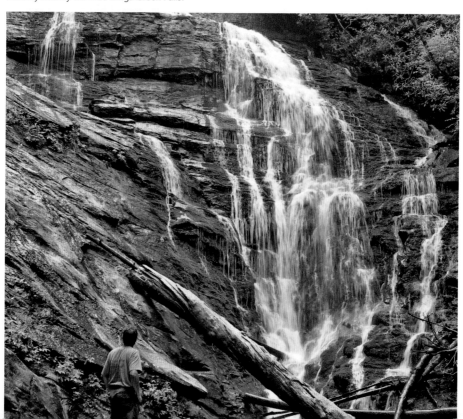

KEY INFORMATION

CONTACT: 864-638-9568,
www.fs.usda.gov/scnfs

OPEN: Year-round

SITES: Not designated, but there is room for 9 tents

EACH SITE HAS: Picnic table, fire ring, lantern post

ASSIGNMENT: First-come, first-served; no reservations

WHEELCHAIR ACCESS: None

REGISTRATION: Not necessary

AMENITIES: Pit toilet

PARKING: At Burrells Ford parking area

FEES: None

ELEVATION: 2,000'

RESTRICTIONS:

PETS: On leash only

QUIET HOURS: 10 p.m.–6 a.m.

FIRES: In fire rings only

ALCOHOL: At campsites only

VEHICLES: In parking area only; no RVs or trailers

OTHER: No trash cans—pack it in, pack it out; campers must carry tents one-third of a mile to site

glade that receives enough sun for grass to grow. All the sites offer maximum privacy, as they are well away from one another. You won't be able to carry enough stuff from your automobile to the campground to use all the space offered at each campsite, although on my visit, one enterprising fellow toted his belongings down from the parking area in a wheelbarrow.

The left fork of the road enters the south side of the river bottom after crossing the clear and cool Kings Creek. Here you'll find more primitive sites: usually just a flat spot, a fire ring, and an occasional picnic table or lantern post. In a nearby flat, just upstream on Kings Creek, a very isolated site backs up against a steep hill for the tent camper seeking the ultimate in privacy. The left fork of the road intersects the Foothills Trail along the river; here, you'll encounter many secluded and flat campsites. Solitude is yours, to say the least.

Burrells Ford is rustic, and, as expected, amenities are minimal. After all, it is within a Wild and Scenic River corridor and borders the Ellicott Rock Wilderness. Two pit toilets are available for your basic comfort. Bring your own water.

To see more of the attractive riverine ecosystem of the Chattooga, you only need to choose whether to go up or down the river. Down the Chattooga is the Foothills Trail. It winds along the river past Big Bend Falls for some 5 miles to Licklog Creek before turning southeast toward Oconee State Park. You can keep south along the river 4.8 miles on the Chattooga Trail to Ridley Fields and SC 28. But first, tune up with a short 0.3-mile hike up Kings Creek to 80-foot Kings Creek Falls, then return to camp.

Upstream and north from Burrells Ford, the Foothills Trail climbs away from the river along Medlin Mountain on its journey to Table Rock State Park nearly 70 miles away. If you stay north along the river, you'll soon enter the 7,000-acre Ellicott Rock Wilderness on the north section of the Chattooga Trail, which leads 4 scenic miles past riverside beaches to Ellicott Rock. This spot was selected in 1811 by a surveyor named Andrew Ellicott to designate the exact location where the Carolinas and Georgia came together. Ellicott chiseled NC in 1811 on this trailside marker. The actual point at which the three states meet is Commissioner's Rock, extending into the Chattooga River a few feet distant. Stand here and you can be in three states at once. Take the short side of the trail to Spoon Auger Falls on your way back.

It takes a little effort to reach Burrells Ford Campground, but you will be well rewarded. The Chattooga deserves its Wild and Scenic status, and the surrounding mountain lands are wild and scenic as well.

Burrells Ford Campground

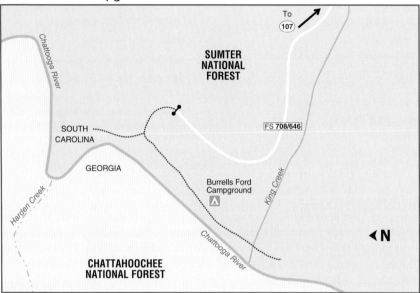

GETTING THERE

From I-85, take Exit 19B (SC 28 West/US 76 West/Clemson Boulevard), and merge onto US 76 West. Drive 11.2 miles; then turn left onto US 123 South/US 76 West/Tiger Boulevard. Drive 9.1 miles; then turn right onto SC 28 West, and drive 15.2 miles. Turn right onto SC 107 North, and drive 10.2 miles. Turn left onto Forest Service Road 708, which becomes FS 646, and drive 2.3 miles to the campground.

GPS COORDINATES N34° 58.297' W83° 06.940'

39

Cherry Hill Campground

Beauty: ★★★★★ Privacy: ★★★★ Spaciousness: ★★★★★ Quiet: ★★★★ Security: ★★★★ Cleanliness: ★★★★★

Cherry Hill is South Carolina's finest upcountry campground.

Cherry Hill Campground is the focal point for the Cherry Hill Recreation Area. And as one of the best national forest campgrounds in the Southern Appalachians, it is a fine place to be. The campground, in the shallow upper valley of West Fork Creek, lies covered with an abundant understory beneath a towering forest of hardwood and pine.

Just off SC 107 is the entrance to the campground. Immediately to the left is a circular turnaround designated as the overflow area. It once was home to a settler, whose chimney still stands just off the loop; a short path leads to the ruins. Four campsites have been carved into the woods there, but you must park on the loop and carry your belongings a few feet to these sites.

The main campground lies beyond the overflow area on a short spur road that descends to tranquil West Fork Creek. Just past the self-service pay station are two sites isolated on their own miniloop. A water spigot is nearby. Three other sites are off the spur road before you reach the main loop, which makes a large oval beside the West Fork.

Miuka Falls on the Winding Stairs Trail

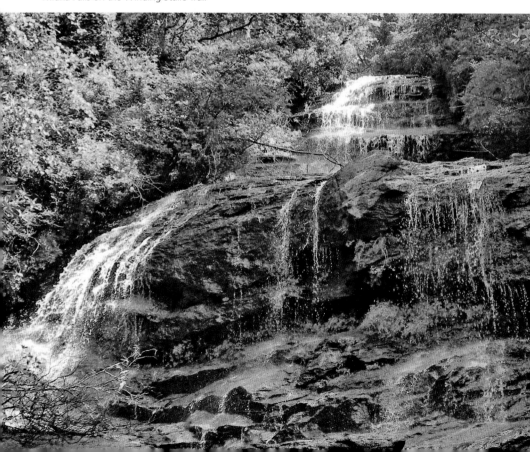

KEY INFORMATION

CONTACT: 864-638-9568, www.fs.usda
.gov/scnfs; reservations: 877-444-6777,
recreation.gov

OPEN: April–October

SITES: 29

EACH SITE HAS: Picnic table, fire pit,
lantern post

ASSIGNMENT: First-come, first-served and
by reservations

WHEELCHAIR ACCESS: Some sites

REGISTRATION: Self-register on-site

AMENITIES: Water, flush toilets, hot showers

PARKING: At campsites only

FEE: $10/night

ELEVATION: 2,250'

RESTRICTIONS:

PETS: On leash only

QUIET HOURS: 10 p.m.–6 a.m.

FIRES: In fire pits only

ALCOHOL: At campsites only

VEHICLES: None

OTHER: 6 people/site; 14-day stay limit;
tents in designated areas only

All the sites along the West Fork are shrouded in rhododendron and are ideal for campers who like deep, lush woods. Four relatively open sites are on the inside of the main loop and offer a generous amount of space for even the most gear-laden camper.

The sites away from the West Fork back against a hill beneath more open woods. Three water spigots are situated throughout the main loop. A clean, well-kept comfort station is located at the north end of the loop; it has warm showers and flush toilets. There are no electric hookups.

Near the comfort station, a small circular drive splits off the main loop. It holds four campsites with large parking areas, apparently designed for RVers, who were the only campers I saw at that spot during my visit. The circle has its own water spigot.

A campground host is stationed at Cherry Hill and keeps the place immaculate and safe. This only adds to the relaxing atmosphere of the area. Just as you get really comfortable, a notion will strike you to venture beyond your folding chair to explore more of the beauty of Sumter National Forest.

And you don't even have to leave Cherry Hill to walk some of the area trails. For starters, try the Cherry Hill Nature Trail. It leaves the campground and makes a half-mile loop among the ferns and brush of the white-pine forest.

The Winding Stairs Trail also leaves from the campground. Follow it down as it switchbacks through an oak forest along the south side of the West Fork. This gentle switchbacking led to the "Winding Stairs" name. At any rate, after a mile, you'll come to Miuka Falls, as West Fork Creek has picked up some volume on its way to merge with Crane Creek.

After the fall, the Winding Stairs Trail veers south to Crane Creek, passing Secret Falls after 2.3 miles, and then returns to West Fork, only to end at 3.5 miles on Forest Service Road 710.

If you want bigger water, the Chattooga Wild and Scenic River is only a stroll away on the Big Bend Trail. The trail starts just across SC 107 from the campground and leads 2.7 miles west into the protected corridor of the Chattooga 0.8 mile upstream of Big Bend Falls. From there, trails lead along the river in both directions for miles. Either way you go, you'll soon understand why this border river between South Carolina and Georgia is protected. The flora, fauna, and tumbling whitewater are yours to appreciate. The fishing's good, too.

Cherry Hill is a great campground in an attractive forest setting. And for 10 bucks, it's a superlative value. Get all your supplies back in Walhalla, because once you're at Cherry Hill, you won't want to spoil your vacation with an early return to civilization.

Cherry Hill Campground

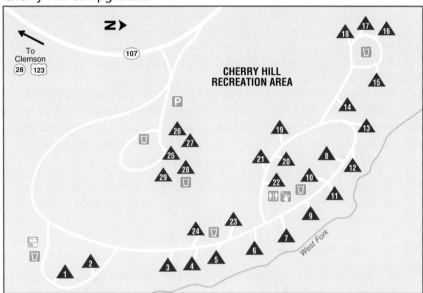

GETTING THERE

From I-85, take Exit 19B (SC 28 West/US 76 West/Clemson Boulevard), and merge onto US 76 West. Drive 11.2 miles; then turn left onto US 123 South/US 76 West/Tiger Boulevard. Drive 9.1 miles; then turn right onto SC 28 West, and drive 15.2 miles. Turn right onto SC 107 North, and drive 8.6 miles to the campground, on the right.

GPS COORDINATES N34° 56.560' W83° 05.280'

40

⚠ Devils Fork State Park Campground

Beauty: ★★★★ Privacy: ★★★ Spaciousness: ★★★ Quiet: ★★★ Security: ★★★★★ Cleanliness: ★★★★

Enjoy walk-in sites that overlook South Carolina's most beautiful lake.

Have you ever seen Lake Jocassee? Others may disagree, but I believe this impoundment to be South Carolina's most beautiful lake. A richly forested shoreline overlooks emerald water against a backdrop of the Blue Ridge Mountains. On the lake's northern shores are the Jocassee Gorges, steep valleys where waterfalls are created by cool, clear streams. Devils Fork State Park occupies some of Lake Jocassee's awesome shoreline, abutted by walk-in tent sites and affording instant water access.

Being a water-oriented park, the campground is, unsurprisingly, near the shoreline. Even better, the walk-in tent sites are close to the lake. The main tent-camping area spurs onto a wooded peninsula extending into the lake, with a paved trail leading down to the campsites. Descend along a rib ridge covered in mountain laurels, oaks, pines, and tulip trees. Sites T1–T8 dip toward the lake but are closer to the parking area. The mountain slope has been leveled at each site. Sites T9–T15 overlook the water and offer a view of the mountains beyond the lake. Landscaping timbers have been installed at the sites and beyond to slow erosion. Sites T16–T19 are too close to one another but overlook the lake; T18 is the best

A paddler's-eye view of Lake Jocassee

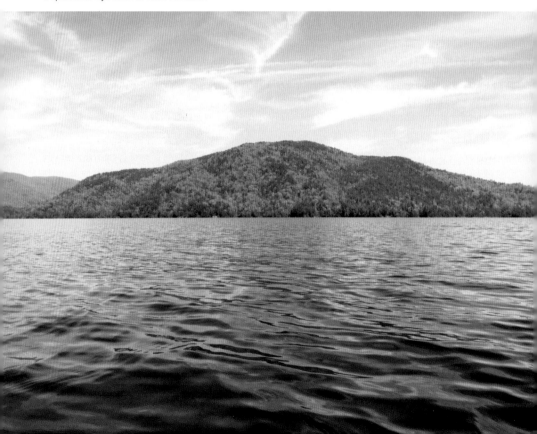

KEY INFORMATION

CONTACT: 864-944-2639, southcarolinaparks .com; reservations: 866-345-7275, reserveamerica.com

OPEN: Year-round

SITES: 25 walk-in tent sites, 59 others

EACH SITE HAS: Walk-in tent sites have picnic table, fire ring, tent pad; other sites also have water and electricity

ASSIGNMENT: First-come, first-served and by reservation

WHEELCHAIR ACCESS: Some sites

REGISTRATION: At park office

AMENITIES: Hot showers, flush toilets, water spigots, laundry

PARKING: At walk-in parking area and at campsites

FEES: $19–$36/night walk-in sites, $23–$45/ night others

ELEVATION: 1,150'

RESTRICTIONS:

PETS: On leash only

QUIET HOURS: 10 p.m.–6 a.m.

FIRES: In fire rings only

ALCOHOL: Prohibited

VEHICLES: No more than 2 vehicles/site

OTHER: No more than 6 campers/ walk-in site

---

of this bunch. Site T20 is closest to the walk-in parking area. The least appealing sites here are T6, T8, and T19, but they are still better than most sites at other campgrounds. A water spigot lies at the beginning of the walk-in-camper access trail.

A second set of walk-in tent sites is accessible from the day-use area, near a playground. Take a short gravel path to reach sites T1–T25, where the woods are more open. Site T22 is near the lake. Sites T23 and T24 are a little too close together. Site T25 has the farthest walk but ends up near some of the drive-up sites in the main campground area. A water spigot is near these sites.

The main drive-up campground has two loops. Trees shade the sites, and ample vegetation screens them from one another. Most have tent pads. Any of these sites will suffice, but the tent sites are far more desirable. And because all sites are reservable, why not go for the ones you like? Reservations are strongly recommended, as the campground fills nearly every weekend from Easter through fall.

This park is fairly small but has two hiking trails. The 1.5-mile Oconee Bells Nature Trail takes you by places where the rare Oconee bell wildflower grows. The Bear Cove Trail makes a 3.5-mile loop and starts at the day-use area. Most recreation is focused on this beautiful lake. You'll see campers swimming near their sites, as no supervised swim area exists. Watercraft access to the lake is made easy at the park boat ramp. If you don't have a boat or you want to get shuttled across the lake to explore some of the Jocassee Gorges, Jocassee Outdoor Center is just outside the park. They have fishing gear and bait, rent motorboats, canoes and kayaks as well as offering shuttles and guided sightseeing, waterfall and fishing tours on Lake Jocassee. Visit jocasseeoutdoorcenter.com for more information.

Lake Jocassee is a gorgeous lake. You can check out all the rivers that feed it from gorges coming out of the mountains—Whitewater River, Devils Fork Creek, Horsepasture River, and Toxaway River. I have explored them via the Foothills Trail, which runs along the north shore of Lake Jocassee, and proclaim them a prize resource of both North and South Carolina. Make a reservation to tent camp at Devils Fork and explore Lake Jocassee; then see if you too think it is South Carolina's most beautiful lake.

Devils Fork State Park Campground

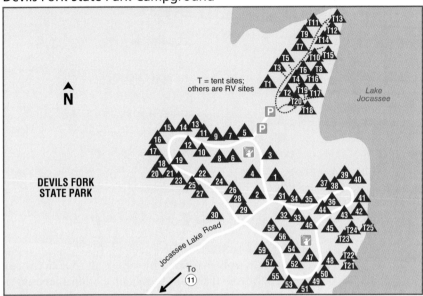

GETTING THERE

From I-85, take Exit 19B (SC 28 West/US 76 West/Clemson Boulevard), and merge onto US 76 West. Drive 11.2 miles; then turn left onto US 123 South/US 76 West/Tiger Boulevard. Drive just 0.4 mile; then turn right onto SC 133, and drive 8.6 miles. Make a slight left onto SC 133/Mt. Olivet Road, and drive 11.8 miles. Turn left onto SC 11 South, and drive 4.6 miles. Turn right onto Jocassee Lake Road, and drive 3.7 miles to the park.

GPS COORDINATES N34° 57.482' W82° 57.233'

41

Keowee–Toxaway State Park Campground

Beauty: ★★★★ Privacy: ★★★★ Spaciousness: ★★★★ Quiet: ★★★★ Security: ★★★★★ Cleanliness: ★★★★★

Cherokee heritage, scenic hill country, mountain lakes, and a peaceful campground make Keowee–Toxaway an outstanding state park.

This area of South Carolina is aptly named the Cherokee Foothills. The Cherokee thrived here long before white settlers ever laid eyes on the land. South Carolina recognizes this, and Keowee–Toxaway tips a hat to native culture in the natural setting of the Cherokee Foothills at this quiet, well-maintained state park.

Tent campers can enjoy the area by day and return to a great campground at night. It is situated on a well-wooded knoll that tastefully integrates campsites with the steep terrain using well-placed landscaping timbers. Shade is abundant beneath the canopy of hickories and oaks, though a relatively light understory somewhat diminishes privacy.

Tent campers have their own separate loop. No loud generators will interfere with the sounds of chirping birds. The 14 tent sites are all spacious and level enough for setting up a normal amount of gear, but expect some seriously sloping topography if you stray from your designated area. That slope, though, allows for balcony-like views into the hollows beyond the campground knoll. The sites on the inside of the loop are less steep beyond

Wild azaleas bloom along the shore of Lake Keowee.

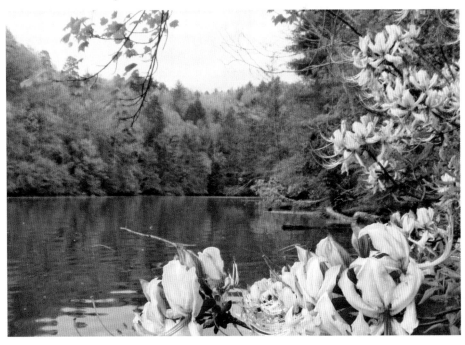

KEY INFORMATION

CONTACT: 864-868-2605, southcarolinaparks
.com; reservations: 866-345-7275,
reserveamerica.com

OPEN: March–December

SITES: 14 tent-only sites, 10 RV sites

EACH SITE HAS: Tent pad, picnic table,
fire ring with attached grill

ASSIGNMENT: First-come, first-served and
by reservation

WHEELCHAIR ACCESS: Some sites

REGISTRATION: Ranger will come by to
register you

AMENITIES: Water, flush toilets, hot showers

PARKING: At campsites only

FEES: $9–$11/night tent sites, $16–$18/night
RV sites, depending on season

ELEVATION: 1,000'

RESTRICTIONS:

PETS: On leash only

QUIET HOURS: 10 p.m.–6 a.m.

FIRES: In fire rings only

ALCOHOL: Prohibited

VEHICLES: None

OTHER: 14-day stay limit

---

their timbered camping area. The tent pads at this state park are among the finest I have seen—they are slightly crowned in the center, allowing for quick runoff during those heavy mountain thunderstorms. This is just one more obvious sign that the campground is well designed.

Another plus is that you'll never have to go far for water. Three spigots are evenly distributed along the small loop. RVers and tent campers share a comfort station located between the two separate loops. Hot showers and flush toilets are provided. Additional features include firewood for sale at the park office and excellent campground safety. In fact, this might be the safest campground in the state. Park gates are locked at night, and the ranger residence is just a stone's throw away from the tenters' loop.

Near the park office is Keowee–Toxaway's centerpiece: the Cherokee Interpretive Center, which recognizes the area's American Indian heritage. During my visit I learned quite a bit about native life before, during, and after the arrival of European settlers, and also about the flora and fauna that inhabit the state park. Visit the interpretive center first for an enhanced appreciation of the historic and natural life here.

Just outside the interpretive center is the quarter-mile Cherokee Interpretive Trail. It winds through the woods and chronicles the evolution of the Cherokee tribe at four informative kiosks, culminating with the story of their removal from their ancestral lands along the infamous Trail of Tears.

Other, longer trails carpet the park. The 4-mile Raven Rock Trail undulates amid the piney hills and hardwood hollows along clear creeks to a rock cliff overlooking Lake Keowee, then loops back via the Natural Bridge Trail to the park's Meeting House. A rock bridge spans Poe Creek along the Natural Bridge Trail. The 0.7-mile Lake Trail leads from the campground down to the shore of Lake Keowee. This park may be only 1,000 acres, but South Carolinians make the most of the scenic beauty packed into the small package.

Lake lovers have two nearby bodies of water to enjoy. Both Lake Keowee and Lake Jocassee back against the Blue Ridge, affording mountainous shorelines. Lake Keowee, the larger of the two, is a warm-water fishery, with bass and bream as its primary sport fish. Anglers will be surprised to find trout in Lake Jocassee's deep, cool waters. Nearby Devils

Fork State Park is on Lake Jocassee and offers good camping as well, with a special section of walk-in tent sites.

Overall, you will find understated Keowee–Toxaway State Park a pleasant surprise. It is ideal for tent campers who want an intimate, well-kept campground with plenty of amenities. The blending of Cherokee heritage and natural beauty was a masterstroke by South Carolina park officials. Don't make the mistake of overlooking this small jewel of the Palmetto State.

Keowee–Toxaway State Park Campground

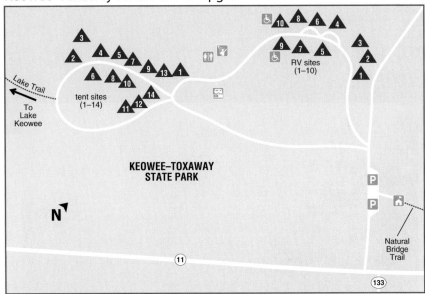

GETTING THERE

From I-85, take Exit 19B (SC 28 West/US 76 West/Clemson Boulevard), and merge onto US 76 West. Drive 11.2 miles; then turn left onto US 123 South/US 76 West/Tiger Boulevard. Drive just 0.4 mile; then turn right onto SC 133, and drive 8.6 miles. Make a slight left onto SC 133/Mt. Olivet Road, and drive 11.8 miles. Turn left onto SC 11 South, and drive 0.1 mile, turning right at the next drive into Keowee–Toxaway State Park.

GPS COORDINATES N34° 56.016' W82° 53.315'

GEORGIA CAMPGROUNDS

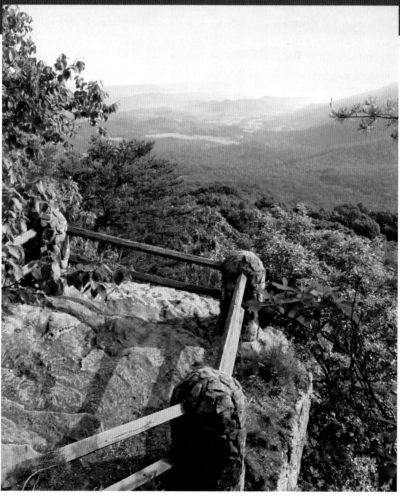

An overlook at Cloudland Canyon State Park (page 142)

Black Rock Mountain State Park Campground

Beauty: ★★★ Privacy: ★★★★★ Spaciousness: ★★★★ Quiet: ★★★ Security: ★★★★★ Cleanliness: ★★★

Georgia's highest state park offers a tent-only camping section and plenty to see from atop Black Rock Mountain.

Black Rock Mountain State Park Campground defies camping stereotypes. It has 44 RV-packed sites with water, electricity, and cable TV hookups, but on a dead-end road on a mountaintop rib ridge is an 11-site, walk-in, tents-only area that complements the rest of the park's sights and activities. The walk-in sites, collectively called Hickory Cove, are the sole reason that this campground is in the book, and these are sites worth your attention.

These walk-in sites are perched on the side of Black Rock Mountain wherever there is a hint of level ground. Some grading and site leveling have been done to make the sites camper-friendly. The mountain setting makes the sites incredibly appealing. Mix in some deep woods with far-off views, precipitous terrain, and a few cool breezes, and you have ridgetop tent camping at Black Rock Mountain State Park.

The main body of seven sites lies north of the parking area. Walk uphill and soon you'll come to the first two sites, set off a bit from the trail for privacy. Thick woods separate all the sites from one another. The next five sites extend farther up the ridge, yet none are

Looking out from Tennessee Rock

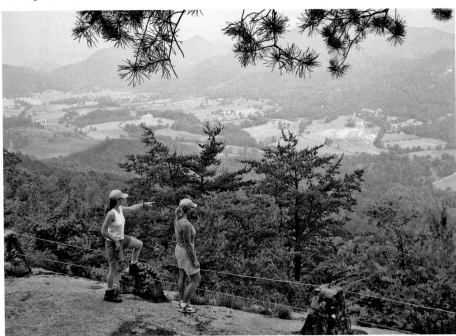

KEY INFORMATION

CONTACT: 706-746-2141,
gastateparks.org; reservations:
800-864-7275, reserveamerica.com

OPEN: Mid-March–mid-December

SITES: 11 walk-in, tents only in season;
44 RV sites

EACH SITE HAS: Walk-in sites have tent pad,
picnic table, fire ring; RV sites have water,
electricity, and cable TV hookups

ASSIGNMENT: May choose preferred site if
available; campground reservations are
non-site-specific

WHEELCHAIR ACCESS: Some sites

REGISTRATION: At campground

AMENITIES: Water, flush toilets, hot showers

PARKING: At parking area for walk-in sites

FEES: $20/night walk-in sites, $30–$34/night
RV sites

ELEVATION: 3,225'

RESTRICTIONS:

PETS: On leash only

QUIET HOURS: 10 p.m.–6 a.m.

FIRES: In fire rings only

ALCOHOL: Prohibited in public areas

VEHICLES: None

OTHER: Park closed
mid-December–mid-March

so far that you can't tote whatever you normally bring on a tent-camping expedition. Just think of it as a little work to achieve the maximum in scenery and solitude. Sites D and E are downhill from the parking area, on either side of their own trail. Sites A and B have their own parking area and are even more isolated than the rest. Still, it's just a short walk back to the comfort station.

The comfort station stands beside the parking area. Inside, you'll find flush toilets, hot showers, and a dressing area for each gender. A water spigot is just outside the building. Ice, soft drinks, and a washer and dryer are back at the main campground. The Trading Post, which is the main campground store, has other supplies. That is the beauty of this setup: you can enjoy all these comforts but still camp in your own rustic atmosphere along with other tent campers.

Five mountains combine to make this the highest state park in Georgia. Black Rock gets its name from the sheer cliffs and outcrops of dark granite, called biotite gneiss. For us that means open views of the Carolinas and Tennessee, as well as Georgia. Due to its high elevation, the mountaintop enjoys the same average summertime temperatures as Burlington, Vermont. Interestingly enough, the Eastern Continental Divide splits the park. Water flowing off the north slope flows into the Mississippi and the Gulf of Mexico; the water from the south slope flows into the eastern seaboard of the Atlantic.

Speaking of water, there's a lake up there too. You can fish 17-acre Black Rock Lake from the bank for bass, bream, catfish, and trout. Swimming is not allowed.

The most popular activity at Black Rock is hiking. Start out on the short Ada-Hi Falls Trail. The trail dips into a cool cove about 0.2 mile on the way to the falls. Because the trail and creek are so high on the mountain, there is not a whole lot of water to work with. Still, the trail will give you a taste of high-country woods.

Next, take on the 2.2-mile loop Tennessee Rock Trail. It swings through varied types of forest and tops out at the 3,640-foot peak of Black Rock Mountain. But the best view is a short way farther at Tennessee Rock. Look both ways at the countryside around you.

We came in late May; the high mountains around us offered varying tints of green as spring made its way up their crests. The valleys below were deep green. The shades became lighter with the rise in elevation. Tennessee Rock is a good place to catch a sunset. Another rewarding trek is the James E. Edmonds Trail, a 7.2-mile backcountry loop that traverses the north end of the park. A highlight of this trail is the view from Lookoff Mountain.

You'll find that Lookoff Mountain is only one of the many sights of this highland sanctuary in the North Georgia mountains.

Black Rock Mountain State Park Campground

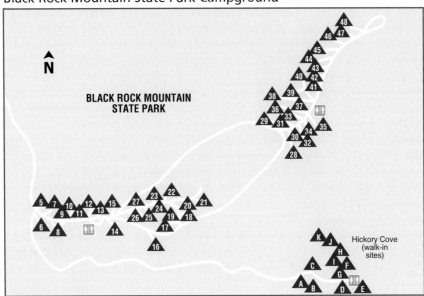

GETTING THERE

From I-85, take Exit 149 (GA 15/US 441/Commerce/Banks Crossing). Turn onto US 441 North, and drive 21 miles. Merge onto US 23 North/US 441 North, and drive 34 miles. Turn left onto Black Rock Mountain Parkway, and drive 1.4 miles to the park.

GPS COORDINATES N34° 55.046' W83° 24.663'

43

Cloudland Canyon State Park Campground

Beauty: ★★★★ Privacy: ★★★★ Spaciousness: ★★★★ Quiet: ★★★ Security: ★★★★★ Cleanliness: ★★★★

Development on Lookout Mountain means top-notch camping and scenic overlooks.

Cloudland Canyon is an example of a state stepping in to preserve a special slice of nature for all of us to enjoy. Sure, Cloudland Canyon is developed to a degree, but part of that development consists of three campgrounds, including a delightful one for tents only. The facilities augment the natural state of things on Lookout Mountain, where Sitton Gulch Creek has carved a gorge on the mountain's western edge, allowing vistas from the rim of the gorge into the lands below.

Atop Lookout Mountain, the waters of Daniel Creek and Bear Creek cut their own gorges into the land before converging to form Sitton Gulch Creek. It is between these two creeks that the East Rim Campground lies. East Rim has 24 campsites spread along a loop meandering through the second-growth pine–oak forest commonly found on the mountaintop. Many of the sites have drive-through parking areas. That means RVs. All sites have water and electrical hookups. A bathhouse with hot showers centers the loop. Many of the park's developed amenities are nearby. This campground may be appropriate for families with young children.

The West Rim Campground is located across Daniel Creek, away from the main section of the park. The mixed forest there is fairly thick, with second-growth trees competing with each other on a slight slope. The 38 spacious sites are spread along two loops. An understory

A view into Cloudland Canyon

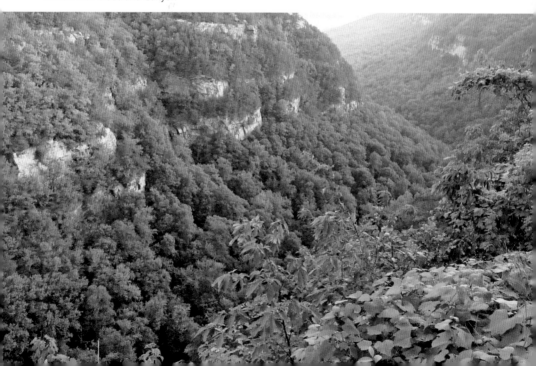

KEY INFORMATION

CONTACT: 706-657-4050,
gastateparks.org; reservations:
800-864-7275, reserveamerica.com

OPEN: Year-round

SITES: 28 walk-in tent sites; 62 tent and
trailer sites

EACH SITE HAS: Picnic table, tent pad, fire
ring; tent and trailer sites have electricity
and water hookups

ASSIGNMENT: May choose preferred site if
available; campground reservations are
non-site-specific

WHEELCHAIR ACCESS: Some sites

REGISTRATION: At campground

AMENITIES: Water, hot showers, flush toilets

PARKING: At campsites and walk-in
parking area

FEES: $20–$25/night walk-in sites, $32–$34/
night tent and trailer sites

ELEVATION: 1,800'

RESTRICTIONS:

PETS: On 6' or shorter leash

QUIET HOURS: 10 p.m.–6 a.m.

FIRES: In fire rings only

ALCOHOL: Not allowed

VEHICLES: None

OTHER: 14-day stay limit

---

of young hardwoods provides plenty of privacy between sites, each of which offers water and electrical hookups. Each loop has a comfort station with flush toilets and hot showers.

The Walk-In Campground is by far the best. Why? First, it allows tents only. Second, it is farthest from the rest of the park developments. Third, it is well laid out in a handsome, forested setting. Park your vehicle in the Walk-In Campground parking area. The sites are spread along a looping footpath on gently rolling terrain. The farthest sites are three-fourths of a mile from the parking area—and are worth every step.

Each site is set off in the woods, providing maximum privacy. There is ample room to spread out your gear. A short trail bisects the campground to access the comfort station, with its hot showers and flush toilets. The atmosphere is of camping in the woods, not of being in a campground with a few trees around.

Cloudland Canyon would not be a state park if it didn't have natural beauty to begin with. Our visit here was particularly scenic. Fall had reached Lookout Mountain. Colorful maples and oaks mingled with the pine trees. The air was brisk. The skies were clear. We knew the views would be inspiring. We set out on the 4.8-mile West Rim Loop Trail, crossing Daniel Creek and skirting the rim of the Daniel Creek Gorge. The trail continued along the main gorge, where overlooks afforded views into the three canyons formed by Daniel Creek, Bear Creek, and Sitton Gulch Creek. We could see the point where the three gorges met, with a blaze of fall color crowning the rim.

The views continued. Below, we could see the town of Trenton. The trail left the canyon rim beyond the last overlook and reentered the mountaintop wood. Eventually we came to the side trail that accesses the Walk-In Campground; we returned to our camp for a hot cup of coffee. Later, we took the short trail to the park's three waterfalls along Daniel Creek. Being autumn, the creek was low on water, yet we enjoyed our walk just the same.

There are still other trails, including the Backcountry Loop. It follows Bear Creek and the east rim. You must find your own overlooks, so be careful. The trail requires crossing a footbridge that is often out from flooding. Inquire at the park office for the status of this trail. Take the Sitton Gulch Trail and climb up the rugged waterfall-rich gorge that is Cloudland Canyon. Mountain. Head to the Five Points Recreation Area where mountain bikers have their own network of trails. Take a guided cave tour, or go a round on the disc golf course. This is primarily a nature lover's place. And at Cloudland Canyon State Park, there is plenty to love.

Cloudland Canyon State Park Campground

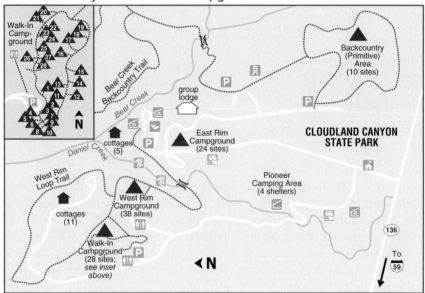

GETTING THERE

From Chattanooga, take I-24 West for about 10 miles; then take Exit 167 (I-59 South/Birmingham). Continue onto I-59 South, and drive 7.6 miles; then take Exit 11 (GA 136/Trenton). Turn left onto GA 136 East/White Oak Gap Road, and drive 0.3 mile. Turn right onto South Main Street, and drive just 0.1 mile; then turn left onto GA 136 East/Lafayette Street. Drive 6 miles; then turn left onto Cloudland Canyon Park Road, and drive into the park.

GPS COORDINATES N34° 49.985' W85° 28.886'

44

⛺ DeSoto Falls Campground

Beauty: ★★★★ Privacy: ★★★★★ Spaciousness: ★★★★★ Quiet: ★★★ Security: ★★★★ Cleanliness: ★★★★

Heavily wooded DeSoto Falls Campground is well located for exploring the central Chattahoochee National Forest.

Where do the names *DeSoto* and *Frogtown* come together? The answer is at DeSoto Falls Campground, which is located along the banks of Frogtown Creek in the 650-acre DeSoto Falls Recreation Area. The sylvan campground provides a good base camp from which to enjoy the scenery of the falls, as well as the nearby Appalachian Trail (AT) and Raven Cliffs Wilderness.

With a campground this nice, it may be hard to tear yourself away. The 24 large campsites are split among two creekside loops arranged beneath a dense forest of deciduous and evergreen trees. This is one of the most densely forested campgrounds I've ever seen; the heavy woods makeseach site seem like an island unto itself and the campground seem more diffused than it really is.

Upper DeSoto Falls

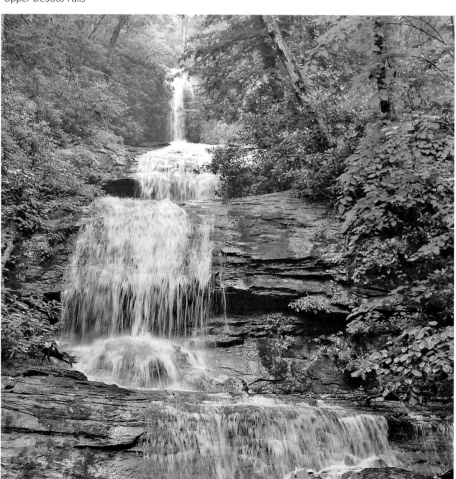

KEY INFORMATION

CONTACT: 706 745-6928,
www.fs.usda.gov/conf

OPEN: Year-round; no water or showers
November–mid-March

SITES: 24

EACH SITE HAS: Tent pad, picnic table,
fire ring, lantern post

ASSIGNMENT: First-come, first-served,
no reservations

WHEELCHAIR ACCESS: Some sites

REGISTRATION: Self-register on-site

AMENITIES: Water, flush toilets,
warm showers, drinking fountains
mid-March–mid-November

PARKING: At campsites only

FEES: $12/night, $6/night winter

ELEVATION: 2,080'

RESTRICTIONS:

PETS: On leash only

QUIET HOURS: 10 p.m.–6 a.m.

FIRES: In fire rings only

ALCOHOL: At campsites only

VEHICLES: 22' length limit

OTHER: 14-day stay limit

The upper loop has a small stream running between the very spacious and private sites, which are separated by thick cover. Four low-volume flush toilets and two drinking faucets are interspersed in the loop. Seven sites border Frogtown Creek but are far enough back to be out of the flood-prone areas. The intonations of the creek can be heard throughout the campground.

The lower loop has three creekside sites; the DeSoto Falls Trail heads west from the loop across the creek before heading north. In the center of the loop is a modern restroom facility with warm showers. Two drinking fountains with connecting faucets complete this deluxe package. The campground has expanded its season and now extends from spring well into fall. Prices are lower during the shoulder seasons.

The primary attractions of this scenic area are the two falls located along Frogtown Creek. Why are they called DeSoto Falls? According to legend, early settlers found a strange piece of armor at the base of the falls. It was supposedly left behind by Hernando de Soto himself as he hunted for gold. Nearby Dahlonega actually did experience America's first gold rush in the 1830s.

The waterfalls of Frogtown Creek are natural treasures. The trail to the falls starts from the lower camping loop. Follow Frogtown Creek downstream 0.2 mile to view the Lower Falls drop some 35 feet onto the rocks below. Return upstream, past the campground, 0.7 mile to the Upper Falls with its four-stage, 90-foot drop. Be cautious as you tread the sometimes slippery trail.

Frogtown Creek and its tributaries offer quality trout fishing. Georgia Game and Fish stocks the stream weekly during the summer. Nearby Waters Creek offers special regulation trophy trout fishing.

Just 1.5 miles up US 129 are Neels Gap and the AT. Either way you hike, you are in for a treat. We went both directions during our trip to the area. The wind blew hard during the 2.5-mile westward pull to the top of Blood Mountain. But the view from the highest point of the AT in Georgia was worth it. The rock outcrop of Blood Mountain, at 4,458 feet, enabled us to see far south into Georgia as clouds floated overhead.

We returned to Neels Gap for lunch and then headed east. First we passed the Walasi-Yi Interpretive Center, the famed hiking and gift shop (the AT actually passes through it). After perusing the unusual ridgetop store, we hiked into the Raven Cliffs Wilderness. The trail wound along the crest until we came to our destination at my favorite peak in Georgia, Cowrock Mountain. With a name like that, it had to be worth hiking 5 miles to see. And it was. The rock-overlaid peak offered views westward into the Boggs Creek watershed and summit after summit beyond that. We returned fulfilled to Neels Gap, then drove to Cleveland and devoured a well-deserved pizza that induced a sound night's rest back at the campground.

Towns Creek Trail (Forest Trail 131) and Dodds Creek Trail (FT 22) are two other pathways that lead into the heart of the 8,000-acre Raven Cliffs Wilderness. If you would like to know more about America's first gold rush, drive 4 miles south on US 129 to US 19, and then drive 12 miles to Dahlonega. The theme of this mountain town is the gold rush. They have some of the typical tourist traps, but also some worthwhile historic buildings and displays.

DeSoto Falls Campground

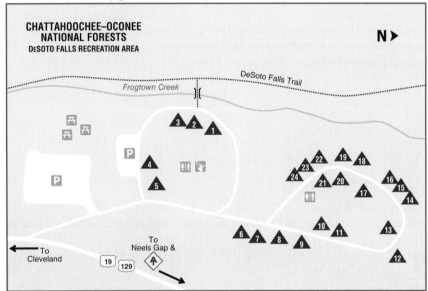

GETTING THERE

From I-285 in Atlanta, take Exit 27 (US 19 North/Cumming). Merge onto US 19 North, and drive about 47 miles. Turn left to stay on US 19 North, and drive 5.1 miles to Dahlonega. Turn right to continue on US 19 North/GA 9 North, and drive 8 miles. Turn right to stay on US 19/US 129 North, and drive 5.3 miles. Turn left to stay on US 19/US 129 North, and drive 4.6 miles; the campground will be on your left.

GPS COORDINATES N34° 42.635' W83° 54.804'

45

Dockery Lake Campground

Beauty: ★★★★★ Privacy: ★★★★ Spaciousness: ★★★★ Quiet: ★★★★ Security: ★★★ Cleanliness: ★★★★

Relax in the highland campground beside the quiet waters of crystal-clear Dockery Lake.

An exceptional campground is set beside a trout-filled lake beneath the shadow of the Appalachian Trail (AT). And that's only the beginning at Dockery Lake Campground. Tucked in a large cove on the southern shore of 3-acre Dockery Lake, this campground is as aesthetically pleasing as the natural mountain surroundings of the Cedar Ridge Mountain Range. The sites are landscaped using native stones with plenty of trees and ground cover that blend in well with the upland landscape. The tent pads are bordered in concrete with gravel pebbles for drainage. Not much leveling was needed, as the slope of the campground is negligible.

The sites are arranged on either side of a one-way gravel road, beneath a pine and hardwood forest with an evergreen understory. Five sites lie directly lakeside; the other six are only yards away but have the advantage of being high enough to overlook the lake. At the campground's end, a retaining wall encloses a small grassy area beside the lake, producing an ideal spot for fishing, sunbathing, or just relaxing.

Serene Dockery Lake is a paddler's paradise.

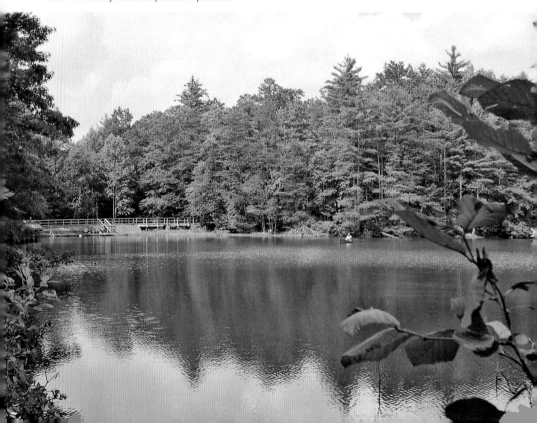

KEY INFORMATION

CONTACT: 706 745-6928,
www.fs.usda.gov/conf

OPEN: Mid-March–mid-December; no water
November and December

SITES: 11

EACH SITE HAS: Tent pad, fire ring,
picnic table, lantern post

ASSIGNMENT: First-come, first-served,
no reservation

WHEELCHAIR ACCESS: Yes, 1 campsite

REGISTRATION: Self-register on-site

AMENITIES: Water spigots, flush toilets

PARKING: At campsites

FEES: $8/night, $4/night November
and December

ELEVATION: 2,400'

RESTRICTIONS:

PETS: On leash only

QUIET HOURS: 10 p.m.–6 a.m.

FIRES: In fire rings only

ALCOHOL: At campsites only

VEHICLES: 22' trailer length limit

OTHER: 14-day stay limit

Two combination water fountains and spigots are positioned around the campground, and a comfort station with flush toilets for each sex stands on the uphill side of the campground. The campground host resides at the campground's center, adding an element of security for visitors. The intimate lakeside environment spells vacation for any camper whose destination is Dockery Lake.

Dockery Lake is fed from the chilly headwaters of Waters Creek, tumbling off the slopes of Jacobs Knob along the AT. The pure water is sufficiently cold to support a healthy population of trout, so it comes as no surprise that fishing is a popular pastime at Dockery Lake. The lake is stocked on a regular basis by the Georgia Department of Natural Resources. Anglers can be found here using a rod and reel lakeside or in a canoe or other small craft. No motors are allowed, however. The 0.6-mile Lakeshore Trail snakes around the lake. Short side trails leading to platforms at the water's edge provide good fishing and lake views. A wooden platform with handrails sits over the small dam. It's a good vantage point for lake enthusiasts to take in the entire 6 acres of the crystalline body of water. The trail is graveled throughout the campground.

The one-way gravel road bisecting the campground leads a short distance to the picnic parking area. Here begins the Dockery Lake Trail, which leads 3.4 miles up to Miller Gap and the AT. Look for deer and grouse feeding in the shadows. After a mile of trail treading along tributaries of Waters Creek, you'll be lower than when you started. The trail climbs for the remainder of its journey to Miller Gap, just shy of 3,000 feet. It's 2.9 miles west on the AT to Woody Gap and GA 60, and it's just over 5 miles east to Blood Mountain, at 4,458 feet, the highest point of the AT in Georgia.

For a scenic overview of the surrounding mountains, drive back to GA 60 and turn right. A quarter mile on your right is the Chestatee Overlook, a cleared area offering a vista of the Chattahoochee National Forest to the east. Another mile up GA 60 is Woody Gap and a view of the Yahoola Valley; the AT passes through the grassy gap. If you need supplies, drive back to Dahlonega.

Dockery Lake Campground

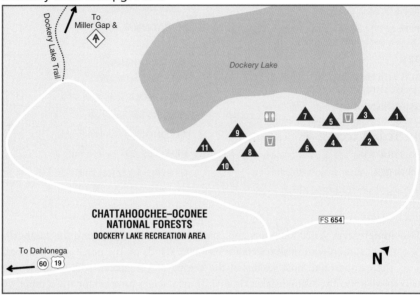

GETTING THERE

From I-285 in Atlanta, take Exit 27 (US 19 North/Cumming). Merge onto US 19 North, and drive about 47 miles. Turn left to stay on US 19 North, and drive 5.1 miles to Dahlonega. Turn right to continue on US 19 North/GA 9 North, and drive 8 miles. Continue straight onto GA 60, and drive 3.7 miles. Turn right at the sign for Dockery Lake, and drive about 1 mile to the campground.

GPS COORDINATES N34° 40.452' W83° 58.540'

46

Fort Mountain State Park Campground

Beauty: ★★★★★ Privacy: ★★★ Spaciousness: ★★★ Quiet: ★★★★ Security: ★★★★★ Cleanliness: ★★★★★

The mysterious rock wall on top of Fort Mountain is just one reason to explore one of Georgia's finest state parks.

Fort Mountain is the site of an unexplained mystery. A strange, serpentine rock wall sits atop the mountain, bounded on both sides by sheer cliffs. The wall, ranging from 2 to 6 feet tall, spans 855 feet and is broken with circular pits at 30-foot intervals, hence the name Fort Mountain. No one is sure who built it or for what purpose, but it is speculated that the wall was some kind of fortification, or was somehow related to religious activities. Either way, it is listed in the National Register of Historic Places. Later, thanks to a donation of land by Atlanta businessman and state senator Ivan Allen Sr. in 1929, forward-thinking Georgians also saw the natural beauty of the area and established a state park.

Autumn colors festoon this trail at Fort Mountain.

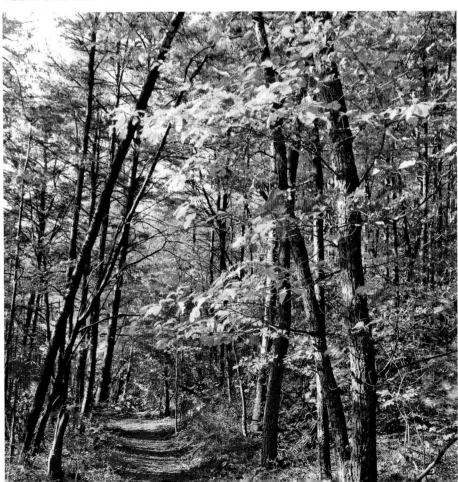

KEY INFORMATION

CONTACT: 706-422-1932, gastateparks.org; reservations: 800-864-7275, reserveamerica.com

OPEN: Year-round

SITES: 4 walk-in tent sites, 62 standard drive-up sites, 6 platform sites

EACH SITE HAS: Walk-in sites have picnic table, fire ring, water and bearproof food-storage locker; others have water, electrical hookups, picnic table, fire ring, and cable TV hookup

ASSIGNMENT: First-come, first-served or by reservation

WHEELCHAIR ACCESS: Some sites

REGISTRATION: At park office

AMENITIES: Water, hot showers, flush toilets

PARKING: At campsites only

FEES: $18/night walk-in sites, $12/night platform sites, $32–$38 other sites

ELEVATION: 2,800'

RESTRICTIONS:

PETS: On 6' or shorter leash

QUIET HOURS: 10 p.m.–6 a.m.

FIRES: In fire rings only

ALCOHOL: Not allowed in public areas

VEHICLES: Maximum 2 vehicles/site

Surrounded on all sides by Chattahoochee–Oconee National Forests, Fort Mountain State Park has two splendid family campgrounds that offer a variety of sites. Set in a hardwood forest on a rolling mountainside, there are 62 shady RV/tent sites, each with water and electricity, and for the more primitive tent camper, 4 walk-in tent sites. In addition, 6 walk-in "squirrel's nests" platform campsites offer a level spot for tents only.

Fort Mountain State Park is peaceful and safe. Quiet hours are strictly enforced. The park gates are locked between 10 p.m. and 7 a.m., and the office is staffed from 8 a.m. to 5 p.m. by accommodating personnel. Three coin laundries and a dump station provide campers with convenience. Get your supplies in Chatsworth before you drive up the mountain, as there are no nearby stores in the high country.

You'll find plenty to do without ever leaving the park. A 17-acre spring-fed lake offers fishing and a swimmer's beach, complete with bathhouse. Tool around the lake in pedal boats or fishing boats, which are available for rent. For the kids, there is a playground and miniature golf course. Scheduled programs, presented by a park naturalist, are offered Wednesday–Sunday during the summer.

Naturally, Fort Mountain has trails. Near the campground, the 1.2-mile Lake Trail loops the lake. Nearby, the Big Rock Nature Trail offers a cliff-edge view off the mountain, halfway along its half-mile loop. Beyond the park office is the 1.8-mile Old Fort Trail, which leads to the 855-foot-long stone wall.

Was the wall a religious site or a defensive barrier to ward off neighboring tribes? Currently, many embrace the wall's possible religious significance.

The wall runs east–west, and many speculate that an unknown tribe of sun-worshipping Indians built it. But Cherokee folklore points to the wall being erected by a group of light-skinned "moon-eyed people" who could see in the dark. (The "moon-eyed people" may have been led by the Welsh explorer Madoc, who according to legend came north from Mobile Bay, Alabama, in the 14th century.) Or was the wall built by Hernando de Soto as a defense against Indian attacks, while he searched for silver and gold? Or was it something else altogether? Explore and decide for yourself.

Take the side trail to the 60-year-old lookout tower, built during the Great Depression from natural materials, then refurbished in the 1970s. The mountains of North Georgia and East Tennessee stand out on the horizon. Hike to the overlook deck west of the stone tower and you will see just how far it is down to the Conasauga River valley below. The really adventurous can attempt the 8.2-mile loop trail that encircles the campground. With such a quality campground situated amid spring wildflowers, summer's lush greenery, fall colors, and winter's clarity, it's no mystery that Fort Mountain State Park is a year-round attraction.

Fort Mountain State Park Campground

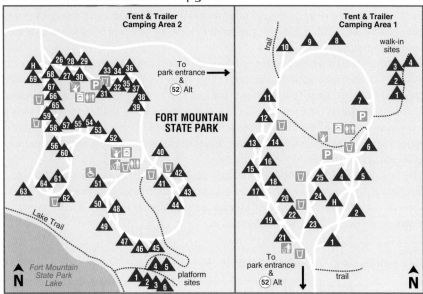

GETTING THERE

From Chattanooga, take I-75 South about 20 miles, and take Exit 336 (Chattanooga Road). Merge onto Chattanooga Road, and drive 0.4 mile. Continue forward onto US 76 East, and drive 5.5 miles. Turn left to stay on US 76 East, and drive 3.5 miles. Turn right onto GA 52 Alt East, and drive 12.5 miles. Fort Mountain State Park will be on your left.

GPS COORDINATES N 34° 45.547' W 84° 41.517'

47

Lake Conasauga Campground

Beauty: ★★★★★ Privacy: ★★★★ Spaciousness: ★★★★ Quiet: ★★★★ Security: ★★★★ Cleanliness: ★★★★

Camp, fish, and hike around Georgia's highest lake.

Set in the rugged western highlands of Chattahoochee–Oconee National Forests, 19-acre Lake Conasauga is a mountaintop oasis adjacent to the 34,000-acre Cohutta Wilderness, Georgia's largest wilderness area. Tent campers will be well rewarded after the long gravel drive that deters all but the most determined RVers. Expect a nearly full campground on weekends. Make sure to bring everything you need—civilization is far away. After you go boating, hiking, swimming, fishing, and wildlife viewing, you will be ready to kick back in the breezy campground.

The campground is located near the lake and divided into three areas. The main campground has 31 sites divided into two loops. The upper loop is on a forested ridge with 12 spacious and private sites. It has several water spigots and a central bathroom atop the ridge with flush toilets for each sex. The lakeside lower loop is shaded by white pine with little understory. Five of the 19 sites are actually lakefront. Those and the other sites offer an appealing view of the clear blue waters ringed in rhododendron. A comfort station and water spigot are located at the head of the loop.

The final five sites sit in the overflow area atop the ridge above the lake. The area has flush toilets but no water, though a short trip to the other loops can amend that problem. The breezes are stronger here, and the area has a mountaintop feel to it. A campground host is located at the largest loop. Recycling stations are in each camping area.

The view from the Grassy Mountain Fire Tower

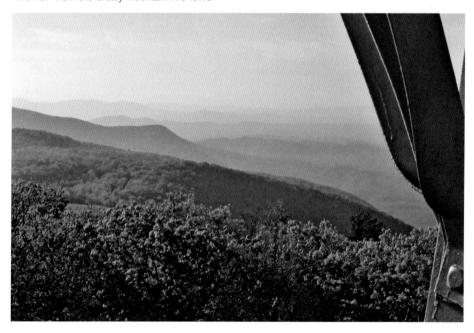

KEY INFORMATION

CONTACT: 706-695-6736,
www.fs.usda.gov/conf

OPEN: Mid-April–October

SITES: 35, including 5 overflow sites

EACH SITE HAS: Fire ring, picnic table,
lantern post, tent pad

ASSIGNMENT: First-come, first-served;
no reservations

WHEELCHAIR ACCESS: Some sites

REGISTRATION: Self-register on-site

AMENITIES: Water spigots, flush toilets

PARKING: At campsites only

FEES: $10 per night

ELEVATION: 3,150'

RESTRICTIONS:

PETS: On leash only

QUIET HOURS: 10 p.m.–6 a.m.

FIRES: In fire rings only

ALCOHOL: Prohibited

VEHICLES: 22' trailer length limit

OTHER: Maximum 5 campers/site

If you find it difficult to pick a site, you will really be hard-pressed to decide what to do first. To explore Lake Conasauga, dammed in 1940 by the CCC, you can take the 0.8-mile Lakeshore Trail, which courses through hemlock and rhododendron along the water's edge. A grassy glade with benches covers the dam. Sit down, relax, and absorb the atmosphere. Or use a canoe or small johnboat and fish for bream, bass, or trout. Only electric motors are allowed. Want to take a dip? Across the lake from the campground is a ringed-off swimming beach. You can reach it from the picnic area or the Lakeshore Trail.

You can start hiking right from your campsite. The Songbird and Grassy Mountain Trails are instantly accessible. Wildlife viewing is made easy by the 0.6-mile Songbird Trail. The Forest Service has cleared small plots along the trail to make a better habitat for the likes of the owl, woodcock, and kingfisher. Beavers have dammed the trailside stream, strengthening biodiversity with their ponds that provide a habitat for numerous amphibians. The 2-mile Grassy Mountain Tower Trail climbs gradually to the 3,692-foot fire tower. From there, you can see the forested Cohutta Wilderness and the Southern Appalachians as they stretch northward into Tennessee.

Just a short distance away from Lake Conasauga are forest roads that circle the southern half of the Cohutta Wilderness. No fewer than six trails lead from these roads into the heart of the Cohutta. Make the most of your adventuring with a map of the wilderness, which can be obtained at the Ranger Station in Chatsworth. The Tearbritches Trail (Forest Trail 9) starts just east of the campground. It crosses Bald Mountain then descends to Bray Field along the Conasauga River. The Conasauga River has a reputation as Georgia's cleanest, clearest waterway. Chestnut Lead Trail (11) drops into the lower Conasauga in 1.8 miles. East Cowpen Trail (30) traverses the high country at the heart of the wilderness. Large trees, wildlife, and good fishing are Cohutta hallmarks.

Conasauga is an area of Georgian superlatives: the highest lake, the cleanest water, the largest wilderness. Come here with high expectations. You won't be disappointed.

Lake Conasauga Campground

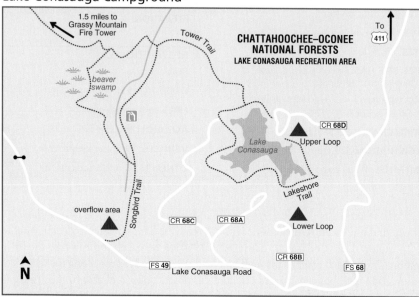

GETTING THERE

From Chattanooga, take I-75 South, and drive about 15 miles; then take Exit 341 (GA 201/ Tunnel Hill/Varnell). Turn left onto GA 201 North, and drive 4.7 miles. Turn right onto GA 2, and drive 12.2 miles. Continue straight onto Halls Chapel Road, and drive 4.1 miles. Turn right onto US 411 South, and drive 2.2 miles. Turn left onto Grassy Street, and drive 0.4 mile then turn right onto Crandall Ellijay Road, and then make an immediate left turn onto Mill Creek Road. Drive 8.6 miles; then turn right onto West Cow Pen Road, and drive 3.2 miles. Turn right onto Conasauga Lake Road, and drive about 0.4 mile to the campground.

GPS COORDINATES N 34° 51.648' W 84° 38.968'

48

Tate Branch Campground

Beauty: ★★★★ Privacy: ★★★★ Spaciousness: ★★★★ Quiet: ★★★ Security: ★★★★ Cleanliness: ★★★★

Enjoy streamside camping and wilderness hiking deep in the Georgia mountains.

Tate Branch, a small, streamside campground, lies nestled far back in the mountains of northeast Georgia. Tate Branch flows through the campground into the unspoiled Tallulah River, which provides a panoramic backdrop for your time here. Near the appealing campground are fishing opportunities, the Coleman River Scenic Area, and the Southern Nantahala Wilderness.

Tate Branch spreads all but five of its sites on a densely forested loop. Thickets of rhododendron produce secluded campsites. A campground host occupies the first site in the loop, next to the pay station, during the warm season. Seven sites lie by the Tallulah River, running about 30 feet wide at this juncture. The next five sites are between the loop and Forest Service Road 70. Two very shady sites sit inside the loop, along with a vault toilet and an old-fashioned water pump. One site is located right off FS 70.

What makes this campground different are the sites in a pine forest across from FS 70. Just beyond a small parking area are four tent-only campsites. Though not that far from the primary campground, the four sites put like-minded tent campers together. Two of the sites lie fairly close to the road, thus requiring very little walking. However, the other two sites sit a little farther back and provide added seclusion. A small meadow lies between Tate Branch and the farthest site.

This sign welcomes you into the Southern Nantahala Wilderness.

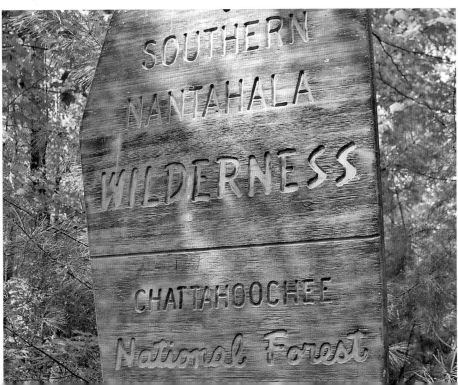

KEY INFORMATION

CONTACT: 706-782-3320,
www.fs.usda.gov/conf

OPEN: Late March–October

SITES: 19

EACH SITE HAS: Tent pad, fire grate,
lantern post, picnic table

ASSIGNMENT: First-come, first-served

WHEELCHAIR ACCESS: Some sites

REGISTRATION: Self-register on-site

AMENITIES: Hand-pumped water, vault toilet

PARKING: At campsites and walk-in lot

FEE: $15/night

ELEVATION: 2,300 feet

RESTRICTIONS:

PETS: On leash only

QUIET HOURS: 10 p.m.–6 a.m.

FIRES: In fire grates only

ALCOHOL: At campsites only

VEHICLES: 22' length limit

OTHER: 14-day stay limit

I stayed at the farthest tent-only site on a day that saw thunderstorms saturate the region. Light from the wildlife opening provided a cheery atmosphere. Yet I didn't stay in my tent and sulk. I donned my rain suit, grabbed a fishing pole, and headed back down FS 70 to the Coleman River Scenic Area. This 330-acre slice of the past is a remnant of the vast, old-growth forest that once cloaked the length and breadth of Southern Appalachia. I cast my lure into emerald pools below cascades that tumbled beneath giant boulders. I had no luck with the fish, but I wasn't paying that much attention as I walked along the Coleman River Trail; I was in awe of the white pines overhead. Drops of rain descended from branch to branch far above me, only to land on the ferns and rhododendron below. The trail dead-ended after a mile. So I turned around and took it all in from a different perspective.

The Tallulah River rose and turned murky after the storm. I drove along its lower reaches on the way to Clayton. I watched the river froth and boil between sizable boulders as fishermen hoped the "stockers" would take their bait offerings. Tallulah River is stocked with trout weekly during the summer. Back at camp, I mustered a fire from wet wood and warmed my bones as fog crept down the river valley.

The Southern Nantahala Wilderness makes for good exploration, also, because it is a rough, rugged, undeveloped area that straddles the Georgia–North Carolina border. This is a great place to hone your orientation skills by exploring old logging roads and unmaintained trails. However, two marked trails will provide a great hike from known position to known position—they also include great scenery. Get the Southern Nantahala Wilderness map at the Ranger Station in Clayton.

Continue up FS 70 until it crosses into North Carolina. FS 70 turns into FS 56 when it enters the Tar Heel State. Shortly after you cross the border, the Beech Creek Trail (378) begins on your right. The trail follows Beech Creek through the wilderness to the high country, passing an impressive unnamed falls as it veers toward Case Knife Gap and its high point. Then the trail switchbacks down to FS 56 and the headwaters of the Tallulah River. Take a short road walk back to your vehicle.

At the end of FS 56 is the Deep Gap Branch Trail (377). It leads 2 miles up the Appalachian Trail at Deep Gap. Just after you enter the wilderness, a short trail leads up a side branch at a falls. Check it out and return to 377. Head east on the AT and come to the

Standing Indian shelter at 0.8 miles. Just 2 miles farther is the top of Standing Indian Mountain. To the east are the headwaters of the Nantahala River and to the west are the headwaters of the Tallulah River. From 5,499 feet, you can look into the Tallulah River gorge. Somewhere down there is Tate Branch Campground. After this hike, you'll be glad to call it home.

Tate Branch Campground

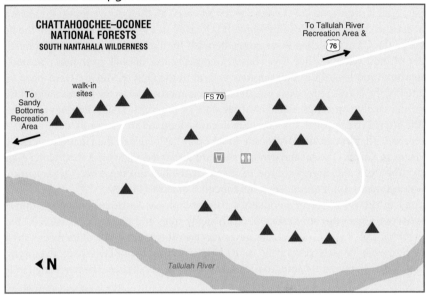

GETTING THERE

From I-85, take Exit 149 (GA 15/US 441/Commerce/Banks Crossing). Turn onto US 441 North, and drive 21 miles. Merge onto US 23 North/US 441 North, and drive 31.1 miles to Clayton. Turn left onto US 76 West, and drive 8 miles. Turn right onto Persimmon Road, and drive 4.2 miles. Turn left onto Tallulah River Road, and drive 4.2 miles. The campground will be on the left.

GPS COORDINATES N34° 57.410' W83° 33.165'

49

Upper Chattahoochee Campground

Beauty: ★★★★ Privacy: ★★★ Spaciousness: ★★★★★ Quiet: ★★★★★ Security: ★★★★ Cleanliness: ★★★★

Camp beside the headwaters of Georgia's most famous river.

Upper Chattahoochee is a favorite campground of mine in Chattahoochee–Oconee National Forests. And it seems the U.S. Forest Service has used all the positive things it has learned in the past to construct this campground. It is located in a long, level cove where the headwaters of the Chattahoochee River merge beneath the high ridges that form the northern border of the Chattahoochee River Basin. Georgia's most famous river flows beyond this campground southward through the state and on to the Gulf of Mexico. Here, deep in the mountains, the Forest Service has integrated the campground into the natural stage of wood, water, and wildlife openings, edged on three sides by the Mark Trail Wilderness.

The attractive campsites stretch out in linear fashion in three sections along a dead-end gravel road. The first group of sites sits in an open flat between the Chattahoochee River and Henson Creek. The second group's sites are dispersed on a short loop along Henson Creek. The third and largest section of sites is at the head of the cove. This arrangement produces a small campground feel, even though there are 34 units.

You can choose whatever woodland setting you please. Some sites are located in open grassy areas. Eight sites are nestled beneath shady trees and require a short walk. But no matter what site you choose, you are never far from the river or one of its feeder streams. Some sites even have stand-up grills, ready for charcoal and your favorite food. Simply put, there isn't a bad site in this campground, only a wide variety of sites. The five, rough miles of

A rocky stretch of the Appalachian Trail in Georgia

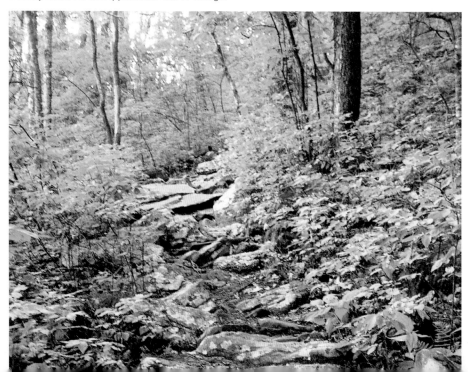

KEY INFORMATION

CONTACT: 706-754-6221,
www.fs.usda.gov/conf

OPEN: Late May–October

SITES: 34

EACH SITE HAS: Tent pad, fire grate,
lantern post, picnic table

ASSIGNMENT: First-come, first-served;
no reservations

WHEELCHAIR ACCESS: Some sites

REGISTRATION: Self-register on-site

AMENITIES: Hand-pumped water,
flush toilets

PARKING: At campsites

FEE: $12/night

ELEVATION: 2,100'

RESTRICTIONS:

PETS: On leash only

QUIET HOURS: 10 p.m.–6 a.m.

FIRES: In fire rings only

ALCOHOL: At campsites only

VEHICLES: 22' length limit

OTHER: 14-day stay limit

gravel road keep this campground from being overrun. During my stay in mid-May, I was the only person at the whole campground.

Three bathroom facilities with multiple low-volume flush toilets are adequately distributed. So are the three hand-pump water sources, which are combination water fountains and spigots. It's easy to recycle in the many recycling bins about the campground. For your safety, a campground host is usually stationed at the heart of the campground.

The short trail to Horse Trough Falls lies at the very head of the campground. The trail leads 0.1 mile to a viewing platform that looks up at the falls. The cascade expands from 2 to more than 30 feet before it gathers again to flow into the Chattahoochee River, just above the campground.

Another popular hike is the 1.6-mile tramp to Poplar Stomp Gap and the Appalachian Trail (AT) on old Forest Service Road 44C. Once on the AT, turn left and hike to the Low Gap Shelter, passing a mature hardwood forest en route. Mountain bikers will like the 7-mile loop ride around the Jasus Creek watershed. The loop starts 4.6 miles below the campground on gated FS 44C.

The Chattahoochee River and its many tributaries offer abundant trout fishing. Low Gap Branch and Jasus Creek provide the angler with miles of remote wilderness, where you can fish far back in thick forest that is normally trampled only by the wild creatures of the Mark Trail Wilderness.

The highlight of my Upper Chattahoochee River adventure was the 38-mile loop drive along the Russell–Brasstown Scenic Byway, which comprises GA 17, GA 180, GA 348, and GA 356. First, I drove out FS 44 to US 129 over Unicoi Gap and then north to the High Shoals Scenic Area. I hiked a mile to the falls—a series of five drops totaling 300 feet. Then I drove to Brasstown Bald, Georgia's highest point. I took the half-mile walk to the viewing tower at 4,784 feet. There I was treated to a 360° view of the surrounding mountains.

On I drove, along streams and on top of ridges, taking in the scenery. I stopped at Dukes Creek Falls, a 150-foot drop down a sheer granite canyon. Beyond the town of Helen was Anna Ruby Falls. It is a double falls, 0.4 miles from the trailhead at the confluence of Curtis and York Creeks. I then returned to the Upper Chattahoochee Campground thinking that maybe the byway should be called the Falls Byway.

That evening, the skies were clear, so after supper I decided to sleep out in the open. Later, I felt a pitter-patter on my face and groggily erected my shelter just in time for a major downpour. The next morning, the Chattahoochee River was roaring beside my camp. I returned to Horse Trough Falls to see a crashing display of whitewater that wasn't present the day before. As I drove out of the campground that morning, I felt extremely satisfied with my experience. And so will you.

Upper Chattahoochee Campground

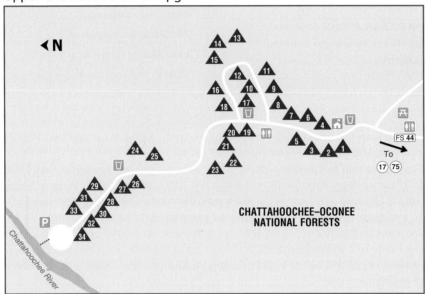

GETTING THERE

From Atlanta, take I-85 North for about 16 miles; then merge onto I-985, and drive 23.7 miles. Continue straight onto US 23 North, and drive 8.3 miles. Turn left onto GA 52 West, and drive 6.2 miles. Turn right onto GA 283 South, and drive 0.3 mile. Turn left to stay on GA 283 South, and drive 2 miles. Turn right onto US 129 North, and drive 7.3 miles. Continue straight onto Appalachian Parkway, and drive 3 miles; then turn left onto US 129 North, and drive 2.1 miles. Turn right onto GA 75 Alt South, and drive 8.1 miles. Turn left onto GA 17 North/GA 75 North, and drive 7.7 miles. Turn left onto Wilks Road/Chattahoochee River Road, which becomes Forest Service Road 44, and drive 4.6 miles to the campground, on your right.

GPS COORDINATES N34° 47.335' W83° 46.897'

50

Wildcat Creek Campground

Beauty: ★★★★ Privacy: ★★★ Spaciousness: ★★★ Quiet: ★★★★ Security: ★★★ Cleanliness: ★★★★

Wildlife, water, and wilderness are just a trail away at Wildcat Creek.

Wildcat Creek Campground is actually two rough and rustic areas located in the 12,600-acre Lake Burton Wildlife Management Area, contiguous to the Tray Mountain Wilderness. A single-lane road with turnouts traces Wildcat Creek and all but eliminates RVs from entering the area. The Forest Service banished roadside camping along Wildcat Creek and constructed these campgrounds to concentrate the impact of human visitors in two areas. The Lake Burton Wildlife Management Area is lightly used except during hunting season.

The two campgrounds are spartan and will put you in the mood for outdoor recreation. Both areas have vault flush toilets and recycling bins. You must get your water from the creek. Be sure to treat or boil it before consuming. Or better yet, bring your own.

Wildcat Creek Area 1 sits just above the confluence of Wildcat Creek and Jessie Branch. Most of the 16 sites are pinched on either side of a loop road circling a creekside flat. However, a few sites rest outside the loop and require a short walk uphill, offering more seclusion and space. Big trees are scattered around the campground, providing ample shade and making up for minimal ground cover. An interesting feature of the campground is the abundance of large rocks placed about the campground by the Forest Service for aesthetics and site delineation. They also make good seats and great tables.

Wildcat Creek waterfall along the Hemlock Falls Trail

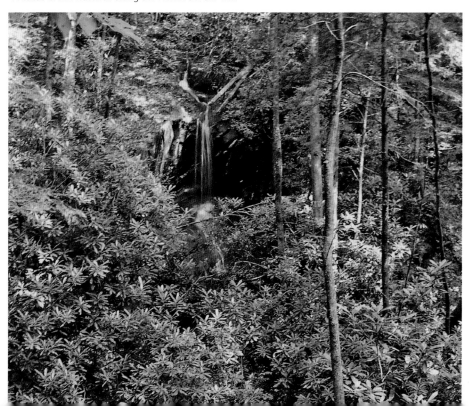

KEY INFORMATION

CONTACT: 706-754-6221,
www.fs.usda.gov/conf

OPEN: Year-round

SITES: 16 in Area 1, 16 in Area 2

EACH SITE HAS: Tent pad, lantern post,
fire pit, picnic table

ASSIGNMENT: First-come, first-served;
no reservations

WHEELCHAIR ACCESS: Some sites

REGISTRATION: Self-register on-site

AMENITIES: Vault toilets

PARKING: At campsites and (Area 1) walk-in lot

FEE: $10/night

ELEVATION: 2,100' at Area 1,
2,400' at Area 2

RESTRICTIONS:

PETS: On leash only

QUIET HOURS: 10 p.m.–6 a.m.

FIRES: In fire rings only

ALCOHOL: At campsites only

VEHICLES: 22' length limit

OTHER: 14-day stay limit

Wildcat Creek Area 2 is bigger and, in my opinion, the better of the two. It has 16 campsites arranged along a figure-eight creekside loop. Large rocks are even more abundant here beneath the tall forest. In addition, the sites here are larger than at Wildcat Area 1. A grassy field created by the Forest Service as a wildlife opening is adjacent to the campground, providing a good escape should you feel closed in by the forest. Just across the creek is the Tray Mountain Wilderness boundary.

For water fun, try fishing, swimming, and boating. Wildcat Creek is stocked weekly during the summer with trout from the Lake Burton Hatchery. Forest Service Road 26 provides easy access to good pools, as well as the Sliding Rock, a popular swimming hole where you can skim over a slippery rock into a cool mountain stream. Be careful, though; those rocks are slippery. The slide is visible from FS 26 before you reach the campgrounds. For true backwoods fishing, follow Wildcat Creek into the wilderness and away from the road. Nearby Lake Burton provides other watery recreation opportunities if you own (or want to rent) a boat.

No trails start from the campgrounds, but you'll find plenty nearby. Just up FS 26 are the Bramlett Ridge and Pigpen Ridge Trails. Bramlett Ridge Trail leads 2 miles into the heart of the Tray Mountain Wilderness, intersecting the Appalachian Trail at Round Top. Follow the AT north and you can loop back to your car from Addis Gap. The Pigpen Ridge Trail leads east 2 miles to Moccasin Creek and a series of waterfalls and slides. You can also access the waterfalls via the Hemlock Falls Trail from Moccasin Creek State Park at Lake Burton. Hemlock Falls is the main attraction but other waterfalls can be seen along the way.

The Wildlife Trail is a gem of a trail. It combines scenic beauty with wildlife openings, enabling you to see the Forest Service's efforts to create a better habitat for the region's fauna. Wildlife openings are man-made clearings containing highly nutritious plants and grasses that are sown for birds, turkey, deer, and other animals. Forest and grassland interface in these openings, producing "edges" where a greater variety of food plants from both environments mix to attract wildlife. Wildlife management is a key element of the Forest Service's multiple-use concept for our national forests.

Wildcat Creek Campground

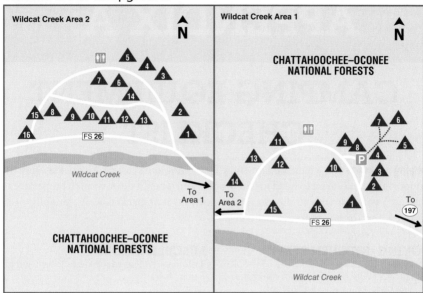

GETTING THERE

From I-85 North, take Exit 173 (GA 17/Lavonia/Toccoa). Turn onto GA 17 North, and drive 13.1 miles. Turn left to stay on GA 17 North, and drive 11.4 miles. Turn right to stay on GA 17 North, and drive 5.1 miles. Turn right onto GA 197 North, and drive 1.1 miles; then turn right and make an immediate left to stay on GA 197 North. Drive 19.3 miles; then turn left onto Wildcat Road/Forest Service Road 26. Drive 3.1 miles to Wildcat Creek Camping Area 1 on your right; Wildcat Creek Camping Area 2 is about 1 mile farther, also on your right.

GPS COORDINATES N34° 49.613' W83° 37.091'

APPENDIX A:

CAMPING EQUIPMENT CHECKLIST

Camping is more fun when you can enjoy it at a moment's notice. You never know when the opportunity may arise to head for the woods, and when it does, wouldn't it be nice to be able to pack your car with all the essentials drawn from prepacked boxes carefully cleaned, resupplied, and stored after your last trip?

COOKING/KITCHEN STUFF
Bottle opener
Bottles of salt, pepper, spices, sugar, cooking
    oil, and pancake syrup in waterproof,
    spillproof containers
Bowls
Can opener
Cooking pots with lids
Cooler
Corkscrew
Cups, plastic or tin
Dish soap (biodegradable), dishcloth, and towel
Dutch oven and fire pan
Fire starter
Flatware
Food of your choice
Frying pan and spatula
Fuel for stove
Lighter, matches in waterproof container
Paper towels
Plates
Pocketknife
Stove and fuel
Strainer
Tablecloth
Tinfoil
Trash bags
Wooden spoon

SLEEPING GEAR
Pillow
Sleeping bag
Sleeping pad (inflatable or insulated)
Tent with ground tarp and rainfly

MISCELLANEOUS
Bath soap (biodegradable), washcloth, and towel
Camp chairs
Candles
Day pack
Extra batteries
First aid kit (see page 4)
Flashlight/headlamp
Lantern
Maps (road, trail, topographic, etc.)
Moist towelettes
Saw/ax
Sunglasses
Toilet paper
Water bottle(s)
Wool blanket
Zip-top plastic bags

OPTIONAL
Barbecue grill
Binoculars
Books
Camera
Cards and board games
Field guides on bird, plant, and
    wildlife identification
Fishing rod and tackle
Frisbee
GPS unit

APPENDIX B:

SOURCES OF INFORMATION

NATIONAL PARK SERVICE

BLUE RIDGE PARKWAY
199 Hemphill Knob Rd.
Asheville, NC 28801
828-348-3400, nps.gov/blri

**GREAT SMOKY MOUNTAINS
NATIONAL PARK**
107 Park Headquarters Rd.
Gatlinburg, TN 37738
865-436-1200, nps.gov/grsm

GEORGIA STATE PARKS
2600 GA 155 SW
Stockbridge, GA 30281
800-864-7275, gastateparks.org

NORTH CAROLINA STATE PARKS
121 W. Jones St., Mail Center 1615
Raleigh, NC 27699-1615
919-707-9300, ncparks.gov

SOUTH CAROLINA STATE PARKS
1205 Pendleton St.
Columbia, SC 29201
803-734-1700, southcarolinaparks.com

TENNESSEE STATE PARKS
312 Rosa L. Parks Ave.
Nashville, TN 37243
615-532-0001, tnstateparks.com

U.S. FOREST SERVICE

**CHATTAHOOCHEE–OCONEE
NATIONAL FORESTS**
1755 Cleveland Hwy.
Gainesville, GA 30501
770-297-3000, www.fs.usda.gov/conf

CHEROKEE NATIONAL FOREST
2800 Ocoee St. N.
Cleveland, TN 37312
423-476-9700, www.fs.usda.gov/cherokee

**FRANCIS MARION AND
SUMTER NATIONAL FORESTS**
4931 Broad River Rd.
Columbia, SC 29212
803-561-4000, www.fs.usda.gov/scnfs

NATIONAL FORESTS IN NORTH CAROLINA
160 Zillicoa St., Ste. A
Asheville, NC 28801
828-257-4200, www.fs.usda.gov/nfsnc

INDEX

ABOUT THE AUTHOR

Johnny Molloy is an outdoors writer based in Johnson City, Tennessee. He has averaged more than 100 nights per year in the wild since the early 1980s, backpacking and canoe-camping throughout the US in nearly every state. The result of his efforts is more than 30 books, including hiking guides throughout the Southeast, tent-camping and paddling guides, and outdoor-adventure books. He continues to write and travel extensively to all four corners of the United States, endeavoring in a variety of outdoor pursuits. For the latest on Johnny, visit his website, johnnymolloy.com.

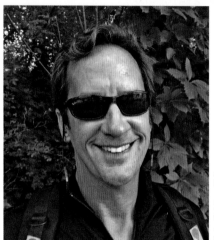

Photo: Keri Anne Molloy